ABOUT THE AUTHOR

Galen Gillotte has been a Solitary Wiccan for more than twenty years. She believes that it is important to honor her hermit self, and seeks silence, solitude, simplicity, and prayer as a way to follow the Goddess and the God, and to maintain balance in her hectic life. Galen resides in southern California with her dog, Sophie.

TO WRITE TO THE AUTHOR

If you wish to contact the author or would like more information about this book, please write to the author in care of Llewellyn Worldwide and we will forward your request. Both the author and publisher appreciate hearing from you and learning of your enjoyment of this book and how it has helped you. Llewellyn Worldwide cannot guarantee that every letter written to the author can be answered, but all will be forwarded. Please write to:

Galen Gillotte
℅ Llewellyn Worldwide
P.O. Box 64383, Dept. 0-7387-0400-8
St. Paul, MN 55164-0383, U.S.A.
Please enclose a self-addressed stamped envelope for reply,
or $1.00 to cover costs. If outside U.S.A., enclose
international postal reply coupon.

Many of Llewellyn's authors have websites with additional information and resources. For more information, please visit our
website at http://www.llewellyn.com

SACRED STONES

OF THE

$\mathcal{G}$ODDESS

USING EARTH ENERGIES
FOR MAGICAL LIVING

2003
Llewellyn Publications
St. Paul, Minnesota 55164-0383, U.S.A.

First Edition
First Printing, 2003

Book design and editing by Karin Simoneau
Cover design by Kevin R. Brown
Cover photograph © 2003 by Leo Tushaus
Interior Illustrations © 2003 by Kerigwen
Spiral Goddess Statue © Abby Willowroot, courtesy of SacredSource.com

Library of Congress Cataloging-in-Publication Data
Gillotte, Galen, 1952–
   Sacred stones of the goddess: using earth energies for magical living/by
   Galen Gillotte
      p. cm.
   Includes bibliographical references.
   ISBN 0-7387-0400-8
      1. Magic. 2. Charms. 3. Precious stones—Miscellanea. 4. Crystals—
   Miscellanea. 5. Witchcraft. 6. Goddess religion. I. Title.

BF1611.G55 2003
133.4'3—dc21   2003055111

Llewellyn Worldwide does not participate in, endorse, or have any authority or responsibility concerning private business transactions between our authors and the public.

All mail addressed to the author is forwarded but the publisher cannot, unless specifically instructed by the author, give out an address or phone number.

Any Internet references contained in this work are current at publication time, but the publisher cannot guarantee that a specific location will continue to be maintained. Please refer to the publisher's website for links to authors' websites and other sources.

Llewellyn Publications
A Division of Llewellyn Worldwide, Ltd.
P.O. Box 64383, Dept. 0-7387-0400-8
St. Paul, MN 55164-0383, U.S.A.
www.llewellyn.com

 Printed on recycled paper in the United States of America

OTHER BOOKS BY GALEN GILLOTTE

Book of Hours: Prayers to the Goddess
Book of Hours: Prayers to the God

To my nephews, David and Steven Hood; their mother and sometime domestic Goddess, Renee Hood; and Louis Francis Gemba, who traveled with me for a time.

CONTENTS

Acknowledgments

I wish to thank the folks at Sacred Circle who attended my class on divination for giving me excellent feedback on my use of stones as a divinatory tool.

Thanks to Louis Gemba for hunting down some hard-to-find crystal and rock specimens, for respecting my need for space, and for forgiving me when I turned into the Red Queen.

Thanks also to Mark Nelson for lending me a lovely specimen of Colorado coal, and to his wife Linda for being so kind.

And finally, thanks to Llewellyn for coming along with me in this new venture, and thanks to those people who worked so hard to make it such a beautiful success: Karin Simoneau for her inspired editing; Kevin R. Brown and Abby Willowroot for taking my vision and turning it into a beautiful cover; Kerigwen for the interior art; and Natalie Harter, who acquired this book—I was her first! Thanks also to the tireless folks in Publicity who send my words into the world that the seekers may find them.

Blessed be.

Introduction

The earth, that solid mass that hangs beneath our feet, has mysteries to share and magics hidden deep within her breast.

Imagine if you will a cavern hidden from the light of day. You enter it carrying a flaming torch and are immediately dazzled by a thousand points of light. Crystals of every shape, size, and color greet you and seem to breathe in the wavering light of your flame. In the silence, you can almost hear them sing.

For thousands of years precious stones, semiprecious stones, and natural crystals have been highly prized and sought after for their beauty and utility. They have been used for personal adornment, to decorate both sacred and mundane objects, in healing, and for the working of magic. Rare gems have been pursued throughout the ages by many, and have even become legend for their size, brilliance, or reputation (usually for bringing bad luck to their owner!). Over time stones acquired attributes and powers, and many ancient beliefs carried over into the twenty-first century, such as: opals are bad luck; red coral will alert one to poison; salt or lava rock may be used for protection; and sunstone will increase sexual potency. Today we have a collection of works that the interested person may access for use in meditation, magic, and healing. However, it is still useful to listen to the stones themselves in order to ascertain their uses and attributes.

Stones may be powerful allies. They hold within their hearts the energy of earth tempered by their own unique constitutions. Each stone is a living being operating in subtle ways, and its energies may be accessed and utilized for a variety of purposes. In this book stones are used in talismanic magic; that is, the stone itself becomes a focus and aid to the completion of a goal. It undergoes purification, consecration, and is imbued with specific energy for the work at hand. The stone literally becomes a touchstone for the magic worked. It is a tool and reminder of the goal one may wish to achieve.

Throughout life we experience many transitions. Change is inevitable, and with each goal we set and each purpose we attain we are changed in some way. Some transitions are guided and nurtured by us; others, such as the loss of a job or a loved one, are thrust upon us. This book deals with those we consciously choose to pursue and offers a set of suggestions on how to achieve them.

Pick up a stone or crystal. Hold it in your hand and *feel* how it feels. Let its energy touch you. Gaze at it, and as you do so notice how the light is either reflected or absorbed by it. Know that it is a key to possibilities, and treasure it as such. Stones and crystals are beautiful of themselves, but there is so much more to them. It is hoped that this book will open up new avenues of thought about these earthy treasures, and that you will find ways to use and cherish them that will enrich your life and engage your imagination.

Part One

The Preparation

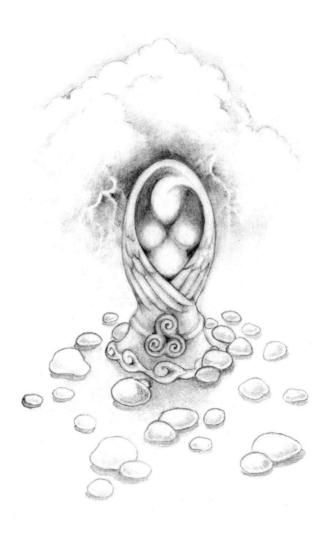

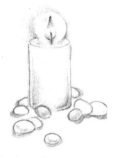

Meditation

*M*editation is that state where the mind is silent, relaxed, and at peace, and the body is at rest. Meditation, unlike relaxation, is an active process, though ideally one should be relaxed prior to engaging in meditation. Results may include a greater awareness, sharper concentration, a sense of peace and inner stillness, a less judgmental or egocentric attitude, and a greater appreciation of the moment. One's consciousness may expand beyond the confines of one's mind to connect with Deity and to perceive the interconnection of all things.

There is no magic to meditation, but there are many techniques available to try. It is not necessarily connected with any religious practice, though it may be found in many religious traditions. Not everyone has the same temperament or needs, thus various techniques have developed to better accommodate the individual. Over the years I have tried several, including: Transcendental Meditation, which makes use of a mantra, or sacred sound, to focus the mind; Centering Prayer, which utilizes a word or phrase to do the same in a Christian context; guided imagery or creative visualization, which engages the imagination and the senses; yoga, which uses breathing and posture; and tai chi, which is a moving meditation that engages both the body and the mind. Other activities that have engendered the meditative response for me include sketching, playing music, chanting, gardening, walking, and doing needlepoint. The focused concentration these activities may require is often enough to release the mind from frenzied, unfocused thought and move it to a still and quiet place.

People engage in meditation for a variety of reasons. Some do so in an attempt to help them deal with stressful jobs or lives. Others may have health problems and use various forms of meditation to help with healing or to cope with physical symptoms such as pain or fatigue. Others do so in order to connect with spirit. Some wish to simply live a more *vibrant* life, becoming more aware and mindful of all they do so that they may better appreciate the moment.

As a clinical social worker it has been my privilege to teach relaxation and meditation techniques to patients and their family members in order to help them cope with physical illness and the various emotional stresses associated with it. Likewise, as a founding member of Sacred Circle, a group of eclectic Solitaries, I have used guided visualization during ritual. Meditation is invaluable for both practical and more esoteric purposes.

In the meditations that are offered in this book I utilize guided visualization. In guided visualization a script is provided that, ideally, engages the mind and the senses for a particular purpose. We engage the imagination and the will in order to achieve a particular result. The meditation encompasses the purpose, affirmation, and spell, and then it is up to you to follow through with some of the practical steps in order to manifest your desired goal. It is a good idea to record the visualization, perhaps with some pleasing background music, so you can really pay attention to and participate in the meditation to the fullest.

Before engaging in the meditation, however, I would like to share some techniques for relaxation, as well as some practical instructions.

RELAXATION TECHNIQUES

It is important to be relaxed prior to engaging in meditation or spell work. The following techniques are simple, not too time consuming, and will dispose both mind and body for the work at hand.

A few simple rules should be followed prior to doing any relaxation or meditation:

- Practice these techniques in a quiet place where you will not be disturbed—perhaps before your altar, if you have one.

- Wear comfortable clothing; avoid anything that is binding or too tight.

- Turn off the television, radio, telephone, and any other possible distractions.

- Before beginning, you might want to take a relaxing bath to let all the stress and tension of the day release into the water and flow down the drain. Use pleasing herbs or some sea salt in the bath to aid with this release.

Once your environment is set up to your satisfaction you may begin at the beginning, with breath.

DEEP BREATHING

Following the breath is in itself one form of meditation, but it is also an excellent technique to use to engender both physical and mental relaxation. Correct breathing is also the foundation upon which all other relaxation, meditation, and prayer techniques or practices are built, so it will be fruitful to practice regularly.

- Go to your special place where you will not be interrupted.

- Turn off the television, radio, and other distractions.

- Sit or lie comfortably. Do not cross your legs or arms.

- Loosen any tight or binding clothing.

- Close your eyes.

- Place the palm of your hand gently on your stomach.

- Now, very slowly and deliberately, breathe *in,* allowing the air to inflate your stomach. You can tell you are breathing correctly if you can feel your palm being pushed out. This will ensure you are breathing *deeply.*

- Hold your breath for a count of three (longer if it is comfortable for you).

- Breathe *out* slowly, allowing your stomach to deflate (your palm will sink down with your stomach).

- Hold the out-breath for a count of three (longer if it is comfortable for you).

- Breathe *in* and repeat the process.

- Do at least five inhale/exhale cycles several times a day to simply remind yourself to relax, or when you become aware you are stressed, or prior to any other relaxation or meditation practices.

Some Things to Note

- Your exhale should take longer than your inhale.

- The key to the exercise is to breathe in and out slowly, and to breathe from your diaphragm (stomach).

- You may breathe in and out through your nose, or in through your nose and out through slightly parted lips, whichever is more comfortable for you.

- If you want, think of the word "relax" as you breathe in; as you breathe out, think of the word "peace." You may use any other word or combination of words that invokes relaxation and peace for you.

PROGRESSIVE MUSCLE RELAXATION

This exercise is for the purpose of relaxing the body. It is easier to enter into meditation when the body is comfortable and free of tension. With practice, this exercise may be comfortably completed in ten minutes. You will begin with deep breathing, which you will continue throughout the exercise. The basic guidelines are below. It would be useful to record them so you can simply listen and relax. Be sure to pause between instructions so you can really experience the muscles becoming free of tension and recognize how they feel when relaxation takes place.

- Go to your special place where you will not be disturbed.

- Turn off the television, radio, and other distractions.

- If you like, listen to a tape that will relax you.

- Sit or lie comfortably. Do not cross your legs or arms.

- Loosen any tight or binding clothing.

- Close your eyes.

- Take a few deep breaths, and begin.

- First, place your attention on your feet and toes. Let all the stress and tension flow out of your feet and toes. Feel the muscles relax.

- Next place your attention on your calves. Feel any tension that may be present just fade away, and let relaxation take place.

- Now become aware of your knees. Let go of any stress you feel in your knees.

- Your body is becoming relaxed.

- Place your attention on your thighs and buttocks. Allow any stress or tension you become aware of to fade away.

- Now become aware of your stomach and pelvis. Notice if the muscles are tight, and just let them relax. Let relaxation flow gently into your stomach and pelvis.

- Your body continues to become more and more relaxed. You may notice a sense of heaviness and warmth in the areas that are relaxed, or you may begin to feel light.

- Now become aware of your back. Let any stress or tension flow away and allow relaxation to take its place. Your back muscles are becoming completely relaxed.

- Now place your attention on your neck and shoulders. If you hold your tension in your neck and shoulders, relax. Let all stress and tension fade away. Your head may fall gently forward as the tension is released, and if so, that's okay.

- You are becoming more and more relaxed.

- Become aware of your chest. Any stress in your chest is now released and relaxation flows in to take its place.

- Next place your attention on your arms, hands, and fingers. If there is any stress present, allow it to melt away. Your arms, hands, and fingers are totally relaxed.

- Your body is relaxed now; your mind is very much at peace.

- Now place your attention on your head and face. Feel your jaw relax. Feel all those muscles of your face relax. Your jaw may open slightly as the muscles relax.

- Your body and mind are now totally and completely relaxed.

- Sit or lie quietly for a while, experiencing a totally relaxed body and peaceful mind.

- When ready, take some deep breaths and slowly open your eyes. Your body and mind will be completely and totally relaxed.

Some Things to Note

- If you lie down while doing this exercise you may fall asleep, and that's okay.

- If you have a particular "problem area" that won't relax, just move on and return to it later. As the body relaxes, these "stubborn" areas will eventually relax as well.

- Different people have different sensations of relaxation. Some find their bodies getting heavy. Some will feel warm. Others will experience a sense of lightness. Others will feel a sinking sensation. There is no one way to feel relaxed, so don't worry about how you should feel. However, you will be aware of feeling deeply and quietly relaxed.

- Enjoy!

Deep breathing and progressive muscle relaxation are good ways to begin the meditations offered in this book. But before getting all relaxed and jumping into the meditations, we need to look at what guided visualization is, and set down some ground rules.

GUIDED VISUALIZATION

Guided visualization is a meditation technique that captures and uses the imagination. The visualization gives the surface mind something to do, while leading it into deeper truths and realizations. Being guided, the mind is allowed to stretch its imagination, but only within set limits. Therefore, it stays focused on a particular objective. The visualization also draws in the senses, engaging the body and keeping it from becoming restless and thus a distraction. Body and mind working together sets up a powerful experience. The visualization will anchor in the unconscious and will continue to process the purpose of the meditation, subtly affecting the self as well as the environment in order to reach whatever goal has been set.

If you have never done guided visualization it is worthwhile to practice a couple of simple techniques in order to help you profit from the meditations in this book. One of them is a candle visualization, and the other is simply called "Orange."

CANDLE VISUALIZATION

- Begin the visualization by completing deep breathing and progressive muscle relaxation. Continue the breathing throughout the exercise.

- Now, in a quiet and slightly darkened room, light a single candle (a taper at least six inches in length).

- Sit before it, about two feet away, and allow your eyes to gaze upon the dancing flame.

- As you watch, your eyes may become slightly unfocused, or even tear a little. Just relax and continue to watch.

- Become aware of the color of the flame, of how the center is darker than the outer part. Notice how the wick may be black and red, and of how the light illuminates the first two or three inches of the candle.

- Become aware of any scent the candle is letting off, either the acrid scent of burning or, if scented, the odor from the candle itself.

- Become aware of how the flame moves.

- Now, after paying attention to these things, allow your eyes, which have become heavy, to close.

- In your "mind's eye," *see* the candle. How do you see an image of the candle? Does it look as it does with normal sight, or are there differences? Can you see the candle in its entirety or only a part of it? Do you see it in color or is it black and white? If you see it in color, has the color changed from the original in any way? Instead of a candle, do you see something else? Something that represents a candle to you perhaps, or something else that gives off light; or even the word "candle" instead of an image, or a flight of colors? Just notice what you see, not what you don't see, as we all "see" things in different ways. Don't worry if you don't "get" anything right away, as visualizing sometimes takes practice.

ORANGE

- Begin the visualization by completing deep breathing and progressive muscle relaxation. Continue the deep breathing throughout the exercise.

- Take a ripe orange and place it before you. Look at it. Notice its color. Notice its form. Be aware of the place where the stem was, and of how the skin is dimpled. Be aware of how the light hits it. Notice how it *looks*.

- Pick up the orange. Notice how it feels in your hand. Is it slightly cool to the touch, or warm? Does it feel heavy and juicy? Does it give slightly if you squeeze it? Is the skin rough or smooth? Notice how it *feels*.

- Now, drop the orange on the table. What does it sound like when it hits the surface? Is it a dull sound? Does it make a "thud"? Notice how it *sounds*.

- Now take the orange and cut it in half. Can you smell it? How would you define the scent? Does the smell make your mouth water? Lift the orange close to your nose and really take a sniff. Does it make you hungry? Notice how it *smells*.

- Now take a slice of the orange and place it in your mouth. Savor the taste. Is it sweet? Sour? Is it cool? Does the juice fill your mouth and trickle down your throat? Is it refreshing? Notice how it *tastes*.

- Now, close your eyes and recall the orange in your mind's eye. Bring back the sensations of sight, feel, sound, smell, and taste. As much as you can, recreate that orange in all of the ways you have experienced it.

- When you feel you have the image, open your eyes and enjoy the orange!

Once again, you may experience the orange in your own unique way. You may see it as if you were looking right at it, or it may appear as an abstract of an orange, or as words or colors, or in some other manner. As with the candle visualization, let the images come as they may.

The previous exercises will help you to experience visualization. Don't worry about whether you are doing it "right," as each person "sees" things in the mind's eye differently. Those who are more visual may be able to recreate a scene or item perfectly, or they may see the scene in the abstract. Those who are more auditory may actually "hear" the scene. Just let your mind unfold the meditation as it will. It should be an enjoyable experience.

Some final guidelines may be helpful. Before engaging in either the relaxation techniques or the meditation you may want to provide yourself with the following instructions in whatever manner works for you:

> During this meditation I will feel safe and secure. No matter what unfolds I can be assured that I am doing the meditation correctly. Outside noises or distractions will not disturb me, but if for some reason I need to be fully present, I simply have to think the thought and I will be. All is well.

The next chapter will deal with magic. Meditation and magic, coupled together, are powerful forces. But always for the good.

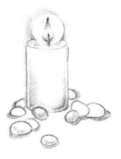

Magic

$\mathcal{M}$agic. The word evokes childhood memories of fireflies dancing in the dark; of fairies living in the garden; of dreams being so real they lapse over into waking time. We blew the fuzz off of dandelions in order to have wishes come true, or wished upon the first rising star. We breathed in magic and were not at all surprised by the wonders we encountered.

Adults lose the sense of magic. For the most part society tells us there is no magic. Disturbed people use "magical thinking" and require medication and therapy to "fix" them, while those less outspoken or flamboyant are simply written off as dreamers. Magic (though not thought of as such) is carefully relegated to religious ritual or created in a Hollywood studio. After all, magic doesn't really exist.

Or does it?

The idea of magic can be very disturbing to those who have had little experience with it, or who come from a fundamental religious background that denies it. There is little understanding of what it is or what it does for these people, and if they think of it at all it is lumped in with "devil worship," something to be feared. Pagans, on the other hand, view it as an energy, neither "good" nor "bad," that is readily available for use in achieving our goals. These goals may include healing, divination, increasing spiritual awareness, bringing prosperity, love, or success into one's life, enhancing skills or unfolding desirable traits, or for other uses as the need arises. Though the energy is neutral, the spell caster may engage the energy for either "good" or "bad" purposes. However, it is hoped that the innate ethical predisposition for the good of the spell caster would prevent him or her from using it in a negative manner, or that the built-in Threefold Law would dissuade the spell caster from doing anything unethical.

Many honored pagans, and some rather disreputable ones, have attempted to define magic. Aleister Crowley—"the Wickedest Man on Earth"—coined what is probably the best known definition: "Magick is the Science and Art of causing Change to occur in conformity with Will" (Crowley 1976, xii). Others have fashioned variations of this. Scott Cunningham, well known in the pagan community, described magic as ". . . the projection of natural energies to produce needed effects" (Cunningham 1988, 19). Elen Hawke, an English Witch and astrologer, states "Life is energy. Magic is energy shaped by the mind toward a specified purpose" (Hawke 2000, 132), and "Magic is shaped by our intentions and works best when we have such need that our whole concentration is focused on a particular result" (ibid., 136). And Starhawk, another well-known pagan author and activist, indicates that magic is the art of ". . . sensing, and shaping the subtle, unseen forces that flow through the world, of awakening deeper levels of consciousness beyond the natural . . ." (Starhawk 1979, 13). I agree with all of the above. Magic is both an art and science that taps into natural energies for the purpose of causing a needed change. As such, magic uses the combined talents of the intellect, imagination, and will to manifest a desired result. In this book you will utilize your own combined talents to make magic happen!

The bottom line is that magic exists. It is a real force. It may be utilized by anyone for any purpose and for this very reason the spell caster must develop a set of ethical standards by which to live. Magic is not lightly entered into, and you must be clear about your use of it. The Witch's Rede (or Law) is a good rule to follow: "An ye harm none, do what ye will," or even Crowley's "Do what thou wilt shall be the whole of the law. Love is the law, love under will" (Crowley 1976, 9). Ultimately you will shape your own world through the use of magic and will have to take responsibility for what you create.

There are various types of magic, but here we are only concerned with talismanic magic. The stone or stones we use become our talismans. They are imbued with the magic energy we raise and thus are objects that will draw to us the result we desire.

Ritual is one form in which magic may be worked. Ritual is a process that usually utilizes certain words, actions, objects, and intentions in order to obtain the purpose for which the ritual is worked. During ritual our consciousness alters from the workaday mundane mindset to an expanded awareness of both inner and outer processes and energies. We raise and connect with the energy called "magic" and wed it to our thoughts, actions, and ritual objects in order to set the magic and achieve our purposes. In this book we use a basic ritual, which will be discussed in the following pages, along with the talismanic objects, affirmations, meditations, and spells to achieve our results.

I recommend that you conduct the meditations and spells presented in the following chapters within a magic Circle. If you have never worked within a Circle, here is a simple Circle cast and Calling of the Quarters you may use, or you may write your own. We work within a Circle in order to contain and concentrate the energy we raise and to keep any distracting energy or entities out. The Circle provides a sphere of protection in which we may meditate, celebrate, or do spell work with complete security. Do not worry about doing it "right"; simply work with the intention that the Circle is cast and the Quarters are called, and it will be so. In addition, other ritual steps follow the Circle cast and Calling of the Quarters.

CASTING THE CIRCLE

There are several steps to casting the Circle that I have delineated here. Before you even start you will want to set up your altar with the items you will need for the working of the spell, such as candles, incense, and appropriate stones. In addition, you will want to include a small bowl of water and another of sea salt (regular salt is okay), and a small bottle of scented oil. The oil may be one of those listed under the "Incense" heading, or you may use rose. The oil represents spirit. You will also need a white candle that represents the light of spirit, and a bunch of dried sage, which will be used for purification of the sacred space. Once everything is set up, you may want to take a ritual bath, using appropriate scented bath salts or herbs. Then you may engage in one or more of the relaxation exercises in order to prepare your mind and body. When all is to your satisfaction, go to your sacred space and begin.

SAGE AND ANOINT

Light the sage, then blow out the flame so it is smoldering and giving off its sweet smell. Waft the smoke about you while saying:

By this sacred smoke I am cleansed.

Take the oil that is on your altar, dip the index finger of your dominant hand in it, touch it to your third eye, and say:

By this holy oil I am blessed.

Now you are ready to go on to the next step.

BLESSING OF THE ELEMENTS

Take each element and make a pentagram-within-circle symbol above it while saying:

Incense:

> Blessed be thou
> O creature of air.
> [Light incense.]

Candles:

> Blessed be thou
> O creature of fire.
> [Light the white candle and then the appropriately colored
> candles for your spell.]

Water:

> Blessed be thou
> O creature of water.

Salt:

> Blessed be thou
> O creature of earth.

PURIFICATION OF THE CIRCLE

Prior to casting the Circle, it's important to purify the sacred
space. Take up the incense, which represents the elements of air
and fire, and walk around the Circle, going clockwise, while saying thrice:

> By air do I purify this sacred space.
> By fire do I purify this sacred space.

Then take the some of the salt and mix it into the water, saying:

> I consecrate thee
> that thou shalt be free
> to bless and purify
> this sacred space.

Then walk around the sacred space, saying thrice:

By water do I purify this sacred space.
By earth do I purify this sacred space.

SCRIBING THE CIRCLE

Now you are ready to cast your Circle. If you have a wand or athame you may use either to scribe the Circle. If not, then use your dominant hand, with index and middle fingers extended. Go to the east and point your hand toward the ground, visualizing a bright white energy extending from your hand to the ground and rising up around you into a sphere as you traverse the Circle. As you walk clockwise from the eastern Quarter, say:

I do conjure this Circle of Power,
strong and bright.
Where death meets life
and sorrow, joy;
where night meets day
and moon and sun embrace,
may light, life, and love
hold sway—
a boundary between the worlds,
beyond the bonds of time
and imagination.
So mote it be.

CALLING THE GUARDIANS

Now you will call the Guardians of the Quarters. These Guardians are called in order to guard and protect the rite, as well as to be witness to it.

Go to the east and say:

Guardian of the eastern gate,
Master of the winds,
wielder of the sharp and terrible sword,

I call upon Thee
to be my guard and protection,
and to witness this most
august rite.
So mote it be.

Go to the south and say:

Guardian of the southern gate,
Master of the flames,
bearer of the sacred lance,
I call upon Thee
to be my guard and protection,
and to witness this most
august rite.
So mote it be.

Go to the west and say:

Guardian of the western gate,
Mistress of the waters,
conveyor of the mystic chalice,
I call upon Thee
to be my guard and protection,
and to witness this most
august rite.
So mote it be.

Go to the north and say:

Guardian of the northern gate,
Mistress of the earth,
upholder of the sacred shield,
I call upon Thee
to be my guard and protection,
and to witness this most
august rite.
So mote it be.

It is nice to have candles at each of the Quarters; yellow for the east, red for the south, blue for the west, and green for the north. You may also scribe an invoking pentacle at each Quarter.

Once the Circle is cast and the guardians are present you will want to invite the Goddess and the God to join in the Circle. Each section has a goddess that directs the spell for that section, and thus you are invoking a particular quality of Hers. But here you will want to invoke *the* Goddess, She who embraces all forms and all attributes. I have included sample invocations for Goddess and God (both, for balance), but feel free to write your own or to speak simply and from the heart.

INVOKING THE GODDESS

O Great Goddess,
rider of the moon,
Thou of the dark and
fertile earth and
Who leads the mysteries,
I request Thy presence
within my sacred Circle.
Bless this work and
make it fruitful.
I honor and thank Thee
for Thy presence here.
Blessed be.

INVOKING THE GOD

Great Horned God,
master of the sacred forest,
Thou Who conveys the sun
within Thine heart and
makes the dream of
rebirth manifest,

> I request Thy presence
> within my Sacred Circle.
> Bless this work and
> make it fruitful.
> I honor and thank Thee
> for Thy presence here.
> Blessed be.

Once the elements are blessed, the Circle is cast, the Guardians are called, and the Goddess and the God are invited into your Circle, you are ready to begin your sacred work. Everything done within the Circle should be for the intent and purpose that you have chosen. Know that the energy you raise will be a potent force to achieve that purpose.

When you have stated the affirmation, completed the meditation, and intoned the spell, you will want to envision the energy you have raised entering into your stone or stones. The stones act as a talisman, drawing to you the fruit of your intention. Each chapter has instructions about how your stone or stones may be used after they are energized and consecrated for their particular purpose.

When you are ready to close the Temple you will want to thank the Goddess and the God for their presence, and will need to release and thank the Guardians and open the Circle.

FAREWELL TO THE GODDESS AND THE GOD

Face your altar and say:

> Thanks to Thee, Lord and Lady, for participating in my rite tonight. To the Goddess and the God I ask Thy blessing and bid Thee farewell. May there be peace and joy between us now and forever more. So mote it be.

RELEASING THE GUARDIANS

Starting at the north and walking counterclockwise, release the Guardians in this manner:

Go to the north:

> Guardian of the north
> I bid thee farewell with
> thanks and bright blessings.
> Go in peace from this Circle.
> So mote it be.
> [Extinguish the candle if one was lit.]

Go to the west:

> Guardian of the west
> I bid thee farewell with
> thanks and bright blessings.
> Go in peace from this Circle.
> So mote it be.
> [Extinguish the candle if one was lit.]

Go to the south:

> Guardian of the south
> I bid thee farewell with
> thanks and bright blessings.
> Go in peace from this Circle.
> So mote it be.
> [Extinguish the candle if one was lit.]

Go to the east:

> Guardian of the east
> I bid thee farewell with
> thanks and bright blessings.
> Go in peace from this Circle.
> So mote it be.
> [Extinguish the candle if one was lit.]

BANISHING THE CIRCLE

Traversing the Circle counterclockwise from the northern Quarter, say:

> This Circle that has
> contained this sacred space
> is now released and undone.
> So mote it be.

EARTHING THE POWER

After any ritual, it is important to earth any stray power that is present. It will also help to settle your energy. So just kneel or sit upon the ground or floor, palms down, and say:

> I release the energy of this Circle into the earth with bright blessings.

Imagine the energy entering into the earth. Then stand and say:

> The Circle is open but unbroken. The Temple is closed.
> So mote it be.

This simple ritual may be used along with any of the sections in order to complete the work of magic you wish to undertake. Feel free to alter or even rewrite the parts if you wish. This is your ritual work, and as long as the basic steps are followed, your own words are as good as any others!

In the next section I will discuss how your stones may be obtained and prepared for use.

The Stones

*C*rystals and stones have become popular in recent years as the interest and acceptability of so-called New Age thought and activities have blossomed. Now polished stones of every type, as well as crystals in the shapes of balls, single- or double-terminated rods, and clusters are sold in every New Age shop and bookstore, through mail order, or over the Internet. However, when considering a stone for use in magic it is best to purchase it from a shop or bookstore. Usually stones are sold individually from trays holding a single type, but not all stones are the same. You must pick them up and handle them until you get a sense that a particular stone wants to go home with you. It is not unusual for a stone to keep "jumping" out of its tray to reach you! By choosing the stone yourself you will begin the bonding process with it.

You should also be aware that some stones may be manmade, so you will want to deal with a reputable source. Stones such as amber and jet have been reproduced in plastic and some turquoise has been dyed to enhance or deepen their color. Try to stay away from these items, as for the most part artificial or altered stones will have little value.

After bringing your stones home and before working with them you will want to cleanse them of any unwanted energy and purify them for the work ahead. There are several acceptable methods for preparing your stones.

BY AIR

You may pass your stone though a cleansing incense such as sandalwood, or smudge it with sage.

BY FIRE

You may pass your stone *above* the flame of a candle.

BY WATER

Since water is a natural purifier, you may hold your stone beneath running water. This may be water from your kitchen faucet, a flowing stream, or an ocean tide pool. Make sure the stone is secure if using the latter two methods. The stone may also be immersed in clear water overnight. Rainwater is great to use for this method. Salt, another natural purifier, may be added to the water if you wish. Some stones, such as opals and turquoise, do not like sudden changes in temperature, so it may be best to avoid the water method with these stones.

BY EARTH

Salt, though a mineral, is also a natural purifier and protective agent. Sea salt is best, but any salt may be used. Bury your stones in salt for a period of time and allow the salt to purify and protect the stones from any negative energy. Or for more delicate stones, you may lay them on top of a bed of salt for the same effect. Throw the salt away after use, as it has soaked up the unwanted energies and cannot be used for anything else.

Another method is to bury the stones in the earth and allow all negativity to drain away. Then the stones may be gently washed.

FULL MOON METHOD

You may put the stone on a bed of salt and place it where the rays of the moon will fall upon it. Ideally the stone should be exposed the night before, the night of, and the night just after the full moon so it may receive the blessing of the Triple Goddess and the benefits of lunar energy. All stones may be cleansed and purified with this method, except those that will be used for solar meditations or magic.

SUN METHOD

Stones to be used in solar meditations or magic may be cleansed and purified using the rays of the sun. The stone may be put on a bed of salt and placed where the sun's rays will bathe it, ideally on a Sunday after the new moon. Doing so will cleanse and purify the stone, as well as charge it with solar energy. Some stones, like the opal, will not fare well with this method, so another method should be used for more delicate stones.

PURIFICATION BY INTENTION

Any stone may be purified through your intention, though I still recommend that one of the above cleansing methods be used as well. Hold the stone in your dominant hand and visualize white, purifying light entering into it. Make a statement of affirmation that the light of spirit now purifies the stone of any negative or unwanted energy.

Once your stone or stones are cleansed and purified they may be kept in a box or pouch until ready for use. You may also handle them in order to become more familiar with their energies, and meditate upon them to gain a deeper understanding of them. Stones and crystals will impart to us their purpose and desire—we just have to take the time to listen to them.

Once in the Circle you will bless and consecrate your stone or stones by passing them through incense, above the candle flame, by sprinkling water and salt on them, and by offering them to spirit as Goddess and God. They will then be ready to be charged according to your will, and may be used to achieve your goal.

The next part offers meditations and magic for a variety of purposes. It is my heartfelt hope and expectation that by working with your stones for your particular goal or goals you will be touched by that magic you once knew as a child. By cherishing your stones and experiencing the magic, may you reach all of your desires, for the good of all an it harm none, so mote it be.

Part Two

The Work

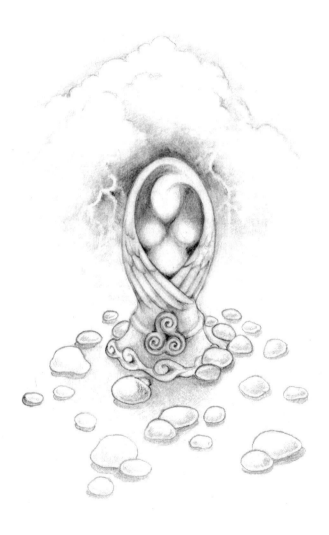

Kuan-Yin: A Spell to Discover Your Spiritual Path

THE MATERIALS

- Amethyst. This may be in crystal form or, if you prefer to wear the gem, a ring, pendant, or several polished beads strung together in the form of a bracelet or necklace will work nicely.

- A purple pouch made of soft but durable material, or a small decorative box (only if you will not be wearing the gem).

THE PURPOSE

We are all spiritual beings. On some level everyone desires to connect with Deity. We know deep down that the reality in which we live is not the only one, and that magic abounds if we can but see it.

There are many spiritual paths that one may walk. Some are "traditional," such as Judaism, Christianity, Buddhism, and Hinduism, to name but a few, and some are new/old paths, such as Wicca, Shamanism, Druidism, Native American spirituality in its many forms, and other so-called New Age offerings.

But how do you choose which is right for you? As we seek to find that path that resonates to the depth of our soul, we are often overwhelmed by the many offerings that exist. The search often takes us from one path to another, leaving us confused and discouraged.

This spell is meant to aid you in your search. It will give you clarity of spirit and help you choose the path that is right for you. If you desire a deeper connection with Deity, but are not sure how to achieve this, you may be assured that this spell will be of help to you.

THE AFFIRMATION

"I walk my spiritual path with joy and confidence."

THE STONE

Amethyst is a stone of the spirit. It may be used to deepen and enhance one's spirituality, and will offer clarity in the realm of spirit. Even its color—purple—is a spiritual color. Violet, one of its shades, is the color of the seventh, or "Crown" chakra, in some systems. Chakras are wheels of spiritual energy that correspond to certain areas of the body. The Crown chakra is placed slightly above the head, but touching it, like a crown. This chakra connects us with the spiritual realms, draws energy from the transcendent and mystical states, and represents self-actualization at its highest level. Amethysts also enhance dreaming and strengthen psychic abilities, both of which are useful for discerning one's spiritual path.

THE GODDESS

Kuan-Yin is a Chinese Buddhist Goddess of fertility, healing, magic, children, and health, but is most well known for Her compassion. Her compassion demands that She hears the cries of the world, and one of Her tasks is to lead others into enlightenment. Because of this quality, She is an ideal Goddess to call upon to help you find your spiritual path.

THE MEDITATION (TO BE DONE IN CIRCLE)

Envision, if you will, a mountain. Its peak is shrouded in clouds and mystery. It is there that Deity resides. There are many paths up the mountain; it is only for you to choose one. You follow the paths with your eyes. Some are fairly easy. Your eyes seek the easy ways, the gentle slopes. There are many spots to stop and rest or to simply enjoy the view. Others are more difficult; they appear to reach the top of the mountain by shorter routes, but also appear almost impossible to walk, with steep switchbacks. At times, there is an abandonment of the path altogether in favor of scaling sheer rock face straight up. Some paths go around obstacles, some over, and others through, with cunningly designed tunnels. You are totally confused: there are too many choices.

As you think about your choice you become aware of a beautiful Lady standing at the foot of the mountain. She is holding a lotus, at whose heart is a brilliant amethyst. She has the most compassionate smile you have ever seen. She holds out Her hand to you. Without hesitation you take it, and together you begin to walk. The path that is yours makes itself known, with clarity and delight, and as it becomes more clear the Lady gives the lotus, with its deep purple heart, to you. It will ever be your guide to your spirituality.

THE SPELL

Go to your ritual place. Set up your altar, cast your Circle, and request the presence of the Guardians. Invoke the goddess Kuan-Yin, and in the presence of All, bless your stone(s) by air, fire, water, earth, and spirit. Sit quietly before your altar and, with stone in hand, engage in the meditation. Keep your affirmation—to walk your spiritual path with joy and confidence—clearly before you. At the conclusion of the meditation, when it feels right to you, stand before your altar and intone the spell, directing energy into your stone(s) as you do so:

Kuan-Yin, Lady of Grace,
grant me a glimpse of
my spiritual place.
Too long I've been
deprived of the light;
show me the path
that will set things right.
So mote it be.

When ready, give thanks to All present for Their assistance. Open the Circle and close the Temple.

You may wear the amethyst on your person, or place it in the pouch or small box and keep it under your pillow. Each day you should hold the gem, keeping in mind your affirmation, and speak the incantation in order to bring your purpose into being.

THE TIMING

This spell is best done on a Monday during a waxing moon. Dawn is an ideal time, as it represents new beginnings.

THE INCENSE

Sandalwood.

THE CANDLE

Purple, for spiritual intentions.

THE PRACTICAL STEPS

- Go to your local library and obtain reading material about the path or paths that seem to call to you. Read up on these to see if their teachings resonate with you.

- Visit various groups and experience their ritual practices in order to see how they "fit."

- Be open to omens: a book that "jumps" off the shelf in front of you; symbols that appear in dreams; unrelated conversations that repeat the same message. Follow your intuition.

THE PRIESTESS SPEAKS

To an acolyte who complains about the frustration of finding her path: "My child, you *are* on the path."

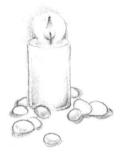

Hestia: A Spell for the Home

THE MATERIALS

• A heart stone, or holey stone, or red garnet.

THE PURPOSE

What do you think of when you hear the word "home"? Does it evoke feelings of warmth, security, and love? Or are memories of home dark and scary? Is home now a place of refuge, of release, of rejuvenation? Do you have a home that you love and cherish, or are you seeking one to call your own?

Home is very often the heart of our lives. We leave our homes to enter a world full of demands, competition, stress, and often ugliness. In our modern age our lives are more hectic than ever in our history, and we sometimes wonder what it's all for. Money? Prestige? Power? These will not of themselves bring happiness and are hollow without an anchor to support them. That anchor is very often home.

"Home is where the heart is" is an old saying, and so very true. Homes come in a variety of forms. Regardless of whether your home is a mansion or an apartment, if you feel a connection and create sacredness within your walls, home can be that place of refuge, of release, of rejuvenation. It can be the place you go to be your true self, without the masks you must wear for others.

This spell is for the home. It is for the purpose of invoking the presence of the Goddess, Who is the center and source of all homes. It invokes Her protection on this most sacred of space so that we may say with heartfelt desire, "Home, sweet home."

THE AFFIRMATION

"I enter my home and become renewed at the source."

THE STONE

For this spell there are three stones from which to choose. As you work with different stones more and more and become comfortable with their properties, you may add others that seem right to you. Those used for love, harmony, and peace would be good choices. But here we focus on protection, for the home should always be a place of security and safety.

- Heart stone. I have discovered that every piece of land that harbors a home or other sacred space has its own heart stone. This is a stone that symbolizes the spirit of the place. It may be easy to find, or it may be buried deep beneath the garden, or even under the house! If you want to try and find this stone you will want to explore your land, leaving no stone unturned, as it were. You may use a divination tool, such as a pendulum, or simply rely on patient awareness to locate it. It will almost thrum when you touch it. It can be any type of stone and any size. If you find it, it will be ideal for this spell. If you relocate to another home, never, ever remove this stone, but return it where you found it.

- Holey stone. This is a stone with a naturally occurring hole through it. It may often be found on the beach or near streams and rivers. Holey stones have been prized for ages for their protective properties and for their connection to the Goddess. People used to hang them from bedposts in order to prevent nightmares.

- Red garnet. This full red stone is ruled by fire. Its color evokes images of the fire's heart. This stone has been used for protection and to repel negativity. It also promotes good health, especially of the heart and circulatory system. The red garnet can be symbolic of the Root chakra and may be used to balance it.

THE GODDESS

The Greek goddess Hestia rules over the hearth and home. Though not a flamboyant goddess, Her color is red and fire is Her element. This virgin goddess was highly revered in Greece and was preeminent in their pantheon. Having Hestia in your home ensures peace and protection. She enters into no disputes, thus encouraging harmony. Her symbol is the hearth fire, which was so important for the ancient Greeks that rituals evolved to determine how a hearth fire may be lit, and it was a sacred duty to see that it never went out. Hestia is the only goddess not represented in any way other than by Her sacred flame. She is an ideal goddess to invoke for the home.

THE MEDITATION (TO BE DONE IN CIRCLE)

In your home, go to your altar and light a red candle. Compose yourself for meditation, and stare into the flame. As you do so envision the source of all hearth fires. Close your eyes and see the fire burning. Stepping out of the flame you see a figure. You cannot see Her clearly and, in fact, She is veiled. Yet you know this is Hestia, goddess of hearth and home. She carries a small lamp that has a red flame burning within. Garnets flash on Her fingers like small fires. You begin to speak but Hestia raises a finger to Her lips, silencing you. Instead, She reaches out and takes you gently by the hand. Envision your home, and see Hestia and you standing by the hearth. If you do not have one, the kitchen stove will work nicely. Hestia reaches out her lamp and the red flame leaps to hearth or burner, there to burn merrily (or if you have an electric stove, to glow with fire's intent). Hestia then leads you from room to room, blessing each one as She goes. You can feel and see the flame of Hestia expanding from Her small lamp to fill your home, without burning anything. You know with certainty that your home is now blessed with Hestia's abiding presence. As She reenters Her flame She leaves behind a sacred stone of blessing for your home.

THE SPELL

Go to your ritual place. Set up your altar, cast your Circle, and request the presence of the Guardians. Invoke the goddess Hestia, and in the presence of All, bless your stone by air, fire, water, earth, and spirit. Sit quietly before your altar and, with stone in hand, engage in the meditation. Keep your affirmation—to enter your home and become renewed at the source—clearly before you. At the conclusion of the meditation, when it feels right to you, stand before your altar and intone the spell, directing energy into your stone as you do so:

> Hestia, goddess of
> hearth and home,
> Lady of the dancing flame,
> consent to enter this
> sacred place.
> Make it holy as
> You are holy.
> Set Your flame ever
> upon its heart,
> that I might know
> protection,
> peace, and love
> within this,
> my home.
> So mote it be.

When ready, give thanks to All present for Their assistance. Open the Circle and close the Temple.

You may place the heart stone upon your hearth, or lacking that, in the "warmest" room of your home. A holey stone may be threaded upon a cord and hung over the doorway you use most. A garnet may be placed upon your altar, or another sacred place, or it may be worn to take the protection and security of hearth and home with you wherever you go.

THE TIMING

The spell is worked best during a waxing moon on a Monday or Saturday. Dusk, the time when we light our lamps, is an ideal time to work this spell.

THE INCENSE

Any incense that evokes the sense of "home" for you, such as cinnamon, cloves, or a particular flower scent. The scent of fresh brewed coffee or baking bread may also be used. (Just don't burn the bread!)

THE CANDLE

Red, for Hestia's passion and for protective energy.

THE PRACTICAL STEPS

- Clean your home! The goddess Hestia likes order. An ordered home is more conducive to positive energies.

- Do a house blessing carrying Hestia's lamp or using the elements. A simple house blessing may be found in the appendix.

- Fill your home with flowers.

- Spend at least some time each day in your home in meditation, allowing the source to touch and renew you.

THE PRIESTESS SPEAKS

The acolyte reverently lights her candle from that of the Priestess and in turn lights the sacred hearth. She then looks to the Priestess for further direction in this most sacred rite.

The Priestess, in silence, points to the kitchen, where dishes are waiting to be washed.

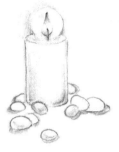

Isis: A Spell to Increase
Magical Abilities

THE MATERIALS

- A collection of thirteen moonstones, to represent the thirteen full moons of the lunar year. They should be drilled so they may be hung on a cord.

- Fine, white cord.

THE PURPOSE

Magic is change brought about by one's will and need. Magic is energy and simply *is*, without being either benign or malignant. Our intent fashions it one way or the other. Magic is not supernatural, but eminently natural and abundant. Magic may manifest itself through prophecy, as in dreams, visions, or intuition. It may be used in divination, attempts to pierce the possibilities of tomorrow. It may be used in healing of body, mind, and soul, or to increase one's creativity, sensitivity, or another attribute one may wish to have. It may be used for such purposes as drawing love into one's life, opening up new career opportunities, for fertility, or other needed intentions. Do not use it malevolently. The Rule of Three states that any intention you send out will return to you threefold, so malevolent intent is unwise, to say the least.

Life may be made better through magic, as long as one is sensible about it. Need, as opposed to want, should be the driving force behind magic-working and spellweaving. As one walks the magical path one eventually learns, through embracing simplicity, that there are very few real needs. However, when a need does arise, magic may help to fulfill it. This spell is for the intention of increasing magical abilities so, when needed, they are more naturally available for your use.

THE AFFIRMATION

"As I spread my wings, magic is mine to direct."

THE STONE

Moonstone is a milky, opalescent stone that is almost wholly transparent. It is connected to all moon goddesses and has been used in conjunction with the phases of the moon. During the waxing moon it is used for active magic, especially love spells, while during the waning moon divination may be done with it. It is also connected with psychic abilities, spiritual development, and freeing the unconscious so one may better know oneself, a prerequisite for working magic.

Since it is so identified with the Goddess and the moon, as well as with psychic and spiritual energies, it is appropriate for use in this spell.

THE GODDESS

Isis, "Great of Magic" and "Queen of Sorcery," spreads Her wings and opens our senses to possibilities. This Egyptian goddess, the fullest flower of all goddess archetypes, is responsible for many things, among them: cultivation, weaving, kingship, government, husbandry, marriage, motherhood, and, not least of these, magic. Isis leads us beyond our conscious levels of awareness to deeper realms and releases us to connect with the self who can wield magic as naturally as drawing breath. Isis is a goddess of the moon, thus, in conjunction with the moonstone, your magical abilities will be heightened, and you may learn to fly.

THE MEDITATION (TO BE DONE IN CIRCLE)

You find yourself in a temple lit by softly glowing lamps. There are symbols painted upon the smoothed stone in vivid colors. One draws you to it. It is a picture of a beautiful goddess, dressed in simple white linen. But upon Her breast is a necklace of gold and jewels. From Her brow springs a headdress—the horns of Hathor cradling the globe of the moon. Her black hair falls around Her shoulders in curls. From Her shoulders sprout the most beautiful wings you have ever seen, many-hued and vibrant. They are out-stretched, tensed for the heartbeat that will send the goddess they support into the sky. You seek this goddess' face; Her kohled eyes gaze back at you, and you fall into Their mystery.

You take flight upon wings of your own; the darkness within your mind parts and secret words of power are given to you. You reach out your hand and contemplate what you find therein: a moonstone, winking back at you. You stare at it, and as you do so it turns into the moon, swallowing you up with Her beauty.

You awaken. The wings are gone but the hidden words of power thrum inside your mind. Thirteen moonstones adorn you, a gift from the goddess of magic, and a reminder that you are now a child of the moon.

THE SPELL

Go to your ritual place. Set up your altar, cast your Circle, and request the presence of the Guardians. Invoke the goddess Isis, and in the presence of All, bless your stones by air, fire, water, earth, and spirit. Sit quietly before your altar and, with stones in hand, engage in the meditation. Keep your affirmation—to spread your wings, directing the magic of your heart—clearly before you. At the conclusion of the meditation, when it feels right to you, stand before your altar and intone the spell, directing energy into your stones as you do so:

> Isis, Great Goddess
> of the night,
> thy moonstone eye
> unblinking in
> my sight,
> grant to me wings
> with which to fly,
> that wonders and magics
> may soon be mine.
> So mote it be.

When ready, give thanks to All present for Their assistance. Open the Circle and close the Temple.

Wear your moonstone bracelet or necklace daily, and sleep with it under your pillow. When doing a magical working be sure to keep in mind your affirmation as you raise power.

THE TIMING

This spell is best done during a waxing moon, close to midnight. It is best done on a Monday, due to its association with the moon, or a Saturday, which is an auspicious time for magical workings.

THE INCENSE

Myrrh.

THE CANDLES

Black. Black is the absence of all color and thus represents all possibilities.

THE PRACTICAL STEPS

- Read! Read! Read! The more you know about what you are doing, the less you have to think about it, and energy will flow more easily. Your local library or bookstore will have many books on magic and related topics.

- Attend seminars and workshops, or join a coven. These days you may find opportunities for learning about magic through your local New Age or Metaphysical bookstore or shop.

- Practice your rituals until they become second nature, thus you will not distract yourself by trying to remember what to do next.

- Meditate before doing any form of magic to determine whether magic is the best solution to the problem. Sometimes it's not. And remember, need, not want, is always a good guide.

THE PRIESTESS SPEAKS

To a frustrated acolyte who feels she's "getting nowhere" with her magic: "Practice makes perfect."

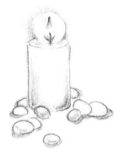

Kundalini: A Spell for Maintaining Health

THE MATERIALS

- A very clear quartz crystal that fits comfortably in your hand.

- A white pouch made of soft but durable material in which to keep the crystal when not in use.

THE PURPOSE

When physically healthy we take good health for granted; when ill, we realize what we are lacking. Indeed, health is the most important and precious thing a person may have. Without it all aspects of our life are affected. When health is poor enough it may, in fact, lead to death.

A crystal or two or three will not magically banish ill health or stave off death. Our life path may lead us where we do not choose to go, through various trials, including illness, for a purpose. If this is the case, our attitude should be one of openness to the lesson. However, the following spell will help you to tune in to your body's needs, and to balance energies before they get too out of sync. Becoming aware of a potential problem and seeking appropriate help is one key to remaining healthy.

THE AFFIRMATION

"I am whole and healthy at this moment."

THE STONE

A clear quartz stone is one of the most powerful all-purpose stones for healing. Since it is clear and reflective it can be used to balance the energies of the major chakras (or energy centers of the body), and can be used in combination with other healing stones to amplify their energies. It has traditionally been used to reduce fever, to treat toothache, to relieve headache, and, when placed on a part of the body in pain, to balance energy and alleviate the pain. To make an all-purpose tonic, leave the crystal in a glass of spring water. This will energize the water. Then take the crystal out of the glass and drink the water.

In this spell the stone is used to balance energies and to allow you to become aware of any areas that may require further assessment.

THE GODDESS

Kundalini is the Hindu feminine life force often portrayed as a serpent. She lies coiled at the base of the spine, and when aroused rises up through the spinal column, energizing the seven major chakras as She goes, until She reaches the crown of the head. There She bursts forth, bringing blissful enlightenment and connection to the cosmic breath. She offers transformation on a variety of levels, but here we are interested in encountering Her aspect as life-force, for with an uninterrupted flow of this energy we may be able to maintain health, or tap into healing energies when needed.

THE MEDITATION (TO BE DONE IN CIRCLE)

You sit in the lotus position comfortably and easily. You are in a stone temple, carved with the images of ancient gods and goddesses. Lush greenery surrounds you. The sounds of birds and other creatures reach your ears. You hear the sound of scales on stone and know a hidden serpent is near, but you have no fear. You hear the sounds of chanting, soft and low, and as you listen, your eyes close and you enter into a light trance. You feel safe and at ease, psychically open. In your trance you see a beautiful snake clothed in the colors of the rainbow coiled before you. Her head is raised and Her enigmatic eyes seek yours. You are not afraid. As the chanting continues, She slowly rises, and as She does you feel points of energy within your body become activated. The chakras are opening, like many petaled flowers: red, orange, yellow, green, blue, indigo, and violet. You feel the cosmic life energy flowing through you, balancing your personal energy and promoting healing if necessary. As the last chakra opens, the Goddess, for such She is, flares Her hood wide and disappears. In Her place is a glowing crystal, reflecting the dazzling colors of your chakras back to you. When ready, you intuitively draw the energy down, closing each energy point one by one, until all the colors lie quiescent within the crystal. You take it in your hand and know that you may use it at any time to balance your energy and draw healing to you.

THE SPELL

Go to your ritual place. Set up your altar, cast your Circle, and request the presence of the Guardians. Invoke the goddess Kundalini, and in the presence of All, bless your stone by air, fire, water, earth, and spirit. Sit quietly before your altar and, with stone in hand, engage in the meditation. Keep your affirmation—to be whole and healthy—clearly before you. At the conclusion of the meditation, when it feels right to you, stand before your altar and intone the spell, directing energy into your stone as you do so:

Kundalini,
cosmic fire,
hidden serpent
of desire,

rise within me
one by one
until the seven
all are done.
Then with exquisite
care, retire
and leave behind
Your healing fire.
So mote it be.

When ready, give thanks to All present for Their assistance. Open the Circle and close the Temple.

Keep your crystal in its pouch when not in use. You may draw out the crystal and either hold it in your hand or place it over the chakras as you engage in the healing meditation at need.

THE TIMING

When drawing healing energy to you, this spell is best done during a waxing moon on a Sunday. Noontime, the height of the day's energy, is appropriate. Conversely, if releasing ill health, it may be done during the waning phase of the moon in the evening, as you imagine the illness receding from you like the tide.

THE INCENSE

Eucalyptus.

THE CANDLES

Green for healing. Red may be added for physical energy. Light blue may be used if the ill health is emotional in nature.

THE PRACTICAL STEPS

- Get an annual physical.

- Listen to your mother and "eat your vegetables!" Try to eat a well-balanced diet to maintain your body's health. Drink plenty of fluids, and if you use alcohol do so only in moderation.

- If you smoke, stop! Organizations such as the American Cancer Society may offer literature or classes, and there are products available through your doctor that can help with the nicotine craving. Hypnosis has also been found to be useful.

- Exercise. Even a brisk walk daily is beneficial. Or look into yoga or tai chi classes. Many forms of exercise may also be used as moving meditations—exercise for the mind as well as the body.

- Sleep your full eight hours. Abundant rest may provide you with abundant energy.

- Play, not only for your body's health, but also for that of your mind and spirit.

THE PRIESTESS SPEAKS

To the acolyte concentrating mightily over her healing crystal and first client: "Stand aside and let the energy *flow!*"

Amaterasu: A Spell to Obtain Clarity

THE MATERIALS

- A good-sized citrine of a rich yellow hue, strung upon a gold chain or fashioned into a ring.

- A yellow or gold box or pouch in which to keep the stone when not in use.

- A handheld mirror.

THE PURPOSE

Life offers us many challenges as we move through the various passages of our lives. In our modern world, which is so hectic with its many demands, we may find it difficult to make decisions about the many areas of our lives that cry out for attention. Issues about relationships, career choices, where to live, what religion to follow, and, ultimately, what is meaningful to us, face us on a daily basis. Decisions are often not clear-cut and can be ringed about by ambivalence, or even the challenge of too many choices. Clarity eludes us and we become stuck, unable to make any move or choice at all, which may lead to depression and even despair. We may simply want to close ourselves off from the world.

This spell is for the purpose of obtaining clarity about a choice that you may be facing. It will help you to find the clarity that resides within, and make it manifest.

THE AFFIRMATION

"My heart reflects the clarity within."

THE STONE

Citrine is a member of the quartz family and is a transparent crystal of pale to deep yellow. Its color is reminiscent of the sun, which sheds its light daily and dissipates shadows. Citrine has been used to disperse negative energy and to engender clarity of thought.

THE GODDESS

Amaterasu is the Japanese sun goddess. She shed Her light generously upon the world until Her brother, the storm god Susano-Wo, who was always teasing Her and playing tricks, destroyed Her rice fields and frightened Her maidens to death. Amaterasu withdrew into a cave, shutting off Her golden light from the earth. The other gods and goddesses, in alarm, tried to lure Her out of the cave, but She refused to budge. Finally the goddess Uzume began singing and dancing, causing the other gods to laugh and carry on to such an extent that, out of curiosity, Amaterasu peeked out of the cave. A mirror had been hung just outside the opening, and when Amaterasu looked out, She saw Her own brilliant self and was transfixed. The other gods quickly blocked the entrance to the cave, and Amaterasu agreed to return Her light and warmth to the earth.

The brilliant light of the sun can symbolically dissipate the darkness within. Clarity may be born from without this light, if we can but accept it. By harnessing our own curiosity we find solutions to seemingly insoluble problems.

THE MEDITATION (TO BE DONE IN CIRCLE)

You are in a dark place. It is so dark that you cannot determine just where you are. You search for a way out but can find no opening. You finally sit on the floor in defeat. Eventually you become aware of a light. It is dim at first, and seems to come from nowhere and everywhere. You notice it getting stronger and stronger until all shadows are banished. You see that you are in a cave. The light now begins to coalesce into a beautiful goddess, richly dressed in gold and white, almost too brilliant to look upon. She holds out Her hands and offers you the gifts She bears. One is a small mirror; the other is a stone that seems to have captured the light of the sun. You accept these gifts gratefully and intuitively know that they may help you through any future darkness. A doorway opens in the solid rock and you exit the cave.

THE SPELL

Go to your ritual place. Set up your altar, cast your Circle, and request the presence of the Guardians. Invoke the goddess Amaterasu, and in the presence of All, bless your stone by air, fire, water, earth, and spirit. Sit quietly before your altar and, with stone in hand, engage in the meditation. Keep your affirmation—that your heart reflects the clarity within—clearly before you. When it feels right to you, open your eyes. Take up your mirror and wear your citrine. Remembering that the goddess has given you these gifts, keep in mind an issue for which you need clarity. Stare into the mirror and allow yourself to gaze deeply into your eyes. Request the Goddess' help in resolving this dilemma. At the conclusion of the meditation, when it feels right to you, stand before your altar and intone the spell, directing energy into your stone as you do so:

> Amaterasu, goddess bright,
> shed upon me Your
> revealing light,

remove this dilemma from
my sight,
while giving me the clarity
to set it right.
So mote it be.

When ready, give thanks to All present for Their assistance. Open the Circle and close the Temple.

Whenever you face a need for clarity, wear your citrine. You may repeat the meditation and exercise as often as needed. Amaterasu may come to you in dreams with an answer, so pay attention!

THE TIMING

This spell is best done during a waxing moon on a Sunday. It may be done when the sun is at its height for maximum beneficial effect.

THE INCENSE

Peppermint or any other "eye-opening" scent.

THE CANDLES

Gold or brilliant yellow for clarity may be used.

THE PRACTICAL STEPS

- Depending on the issue about which you need clarity, you may be able to obtain information. Talk to people who may have expertise in the area. Go to the library and check out reading material. The more you know about an issue the more confident you may feel in making a decision.

- Some issues may not be resolved intellectually with study and research, such as issues of the heart. If so, you may want to take a class about assertiveness training or communication techniques. The better we communicate the easier it is to resolve issues of the heart. Seeing a licensed therapist for counseling may also be helpful.

• Meditate upon your problem and set the unconscious to work on it. Dreams, or the images found in clouds, in a flickering fire, or flowing water may often give you insights that enable you to work through a problem.

• Keep a journal. Sometimes clarity comes from the act of writing out a problem, then rereading what you have written. The answer may seem obvious after such an exercise.

THE PRIESTESS SPEAKS

The acolyte seeks clarity about an issue. She has spent days within her cell, thinking furiously and muttering to herself.

The Priestess enters the cell, flinging open the door and window, allowing the new light of day to enter in.

The acolyte, startled, has an "ah-ha" experience on the spot.

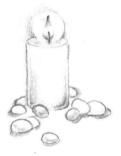

Aphrodite: A Spell to Draw Love into Your Life

THE MATERIALS

- Rose quartz beads, drilled for stringing.

- Rose quartz heart, drilled for stringing.

- Fine cord.

- A rose-colored pouch of soft but durable material in which to keep your stones when not in use.

THE PURPOSE

One of the greatest privileges in our lives is to love and be loved. Life may be satisfying and full without deep relationships, but it very seldom finds itself content; there is always *something* missing. Love allows us to become the best that we can be; it reveals what we lack, and fills that emptiness with itself. The giving and receiving of love calls forth both generosity and the ability to be open and receptive. It is the humble heart that is able to receive. The more we give, the more we have. Love cannot of itself make us happy, but it is the source of all happiness as long as we let it flow and do not try to horde or hold on to it. Trying to hold on to it is like trying to grasp water; it escapes even as we close our fingers.

Having someone to love opens up possibilities and calls forth our strengths and vulnerabilities. We are fully complete and alive only if we can participate in loving and being loved by another. For some this takes an entire lifetime to *get;* for others, "love at first sight" is a real experience.

This spell is for the purpose of drawing love into your life. It is a "generic" spell; that is, it is not for the purpose of making a specific person fall in love with you. Manipulating another's feelings and actions is abhorrent to magic and almost always ends in disaster. Use this spell when you feel the need for love, and let it unfold as it will.

THE AFFIRMATION

"I am a loving and loveable person."

THE STONE

Rose quartz is a member of the quartz family, and may be a pale to deep pink or rose color. It may be translucent to opaque, used in natural crystal form or shaped and polished. This crystal has the effect of drawing love into one's life and opening the heart chakra. It is especially good for self-forgiveness and self-love. One cannot love or be loved by another until first loving and accepting, or treasuring, oneself.

THE GODDESS

Aphrodite is the Greek goddess of passionate love. She was born when the severed genitals of Her father Kronos were cast into the sea. From this rather grim beginning She arose from the foam, glorious and golden. She is a transformative goddess, as one might expect, for love does transform us. Her realm is of the moment, ephemeral, and She is not a goddess to invoke if domestic bliss is sought. However, if you already have a lover She may be invoked to "spice up" your love life!

Aphrodite is multifaceted and powerful. She will infuse any relationship with passion, and Her nature is sensual and uninhibited. She may be invoked to lead you to that self that longs to embrace the moment and plunge into the depths of passion. Be aware that if you do choose to invoke Her, She works quickly and you may be overwhelmed by Her response!

THE MEDITATION (TO BE DONE IN CIRCLE)

You rise from the sea, naked and glorious, the sea foam forming a lacey gown, shells and precious stones adorning your hair. A gentle wind blows you to an island, where a temple awaits you. You step upon the beach, and where you walk flowers spring up in your wake. You enter the temple and find yourself before a full-length mirror. There you see a reflection of yourself—but not yourself alone. Aphrodite stares back at you. Her eyes are glorious, Her hair is alive, and Her body is perfect. Then, with a shimmer, She is gone, and you see yourself as She sees you: beautiful, strong, passionate, amazing—just as you are. You hug yourself in joy and acceptance. Then you notice a small gold casket at the foot of the mirror. You bend down to open it and find a necklace of polished stones in the shape of the moon, with a heart at the center. A rose light glows within the stones. You place the necklace around your neck and as you do you ask the Goddess to send you a lover worthy of you. The pink heart grows warm to your touch and you know that Aphrodite has heard, and granted, your desire. Glancing in the mirror again you catch a glimpse of your future lover. Now it is up to you to accept him or her.

THE SPELL

Go to your ritual place. Set up your altar, cast your Circle, and request the presence of the Guardians. Invoke the goddess Aphrodite, and in the presence of All, bless your stones by air, fire, water, earth, and spirit. Sit quietly before your altar and, with stones in hand, engage in the meditation. Keep your affirmation—that you are a loving and lovable person—clearly before you. At the conclusion of the meditation, when it feels right to you, stand before your altar and intone the spell, directing energy into your stones as you do so:

> Aphrodite,
> goddess of sea foam,
> of perfumed pleasure,
> I call upon Thee.
> In strength and beauty
> am I formed;
> for passion am
> I fashioned.
> Desire drips from my fingers.
> As Thy Priestess I seek love;
> like a butterfly or dragon
> I spread my wings and
> fling myself into love's heart.
> Great Goddess, send love to me,
> that I might drown at last
> in an eternity of bliss.
> So mote it be.

When ready, give thanks to All present for Their assistance. Open the Circle and close the Temple.

You may wear the rose quartz necklace whenever you feel the need for love. Wear it as you go out and about in the world, as it will send out the right "vibes" to attract love to you.

THE TIMING

This spell is best done during a waxing moon on a Friday. Dawn or dusk, both of which are times of transformation, would be ideal.

THE INCENSE

Rose.

THE CANDLES

Pink for love and friendship combined with red for physical love and passion.

THE PRACTICAL STEPS

- Join a club. Take a class. Become involved with a volunteer organization. Enter into activities that will bring you into contact with others (throw out those fairy tales about the knight coming to *you!*).

- Do something nice for yourself: go to a spa; get your hair done; splurge on some new clothes.

- Learn something new every month. Feelings of accomplishment often make us feel good about ourselves and give us a sense of confidence and self-worth.

- Keep a journal or Affirmation Book and write down something nice about yourself every day. Repeat one or more of the affirmations to yourself in the morning as you gaze into your mirror.

THE PRIESTESS SPEAKS

To the acolyte tottering about on six-inch heels, perfumed and painted within an inch of her life: "I think what we're trying to unearth is your *inner* beauty!"

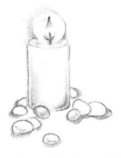

Hera: A Spell for Fidelity

THE MATERIALS

- Lapis lazuli. Ideally, it should be cut, polished, and set into two rings.

THE PURPOSE

Marriage or any committed relationship is comprised of many elements; love, certainly, and liking. Ideally, your partner should be your best friend. Trust and respect are important, as are loyalty and (old-fashioned though it is) devotion. Physical and emotional intimacy and passion should be present, which includes being attracted to your mate and appreciating and admiring him or her. The ability and willingness to communicate openly and honestly should also be present. Compassion and empathy for one's mate is also necessary. And let us not forget a sense of humor and laughter, which includes the ability to laugh at oneself at times! Fidelity, or faithfulness—not only of body, but also of heart, mind, and spirit—is also an important and indispensable ingredient of a good relationship.

From fidelity, trust and respect flows. Fidelity engenders devotion. For many, fidelity is a turn-on and keeps the physical and emotional connection healthy and strong. Fidelity is an agreement to be true to personal and/or religious or social promises, or vows made between two people who choose to share their lives together.

This spell is for the purpose of strengthening the bond of fidelity that already exists between a couple. It is ideally worked with both people present, participating in the meditation and spell together.

THE AFFIRMATION

"Our bond of fidelity is passionate and deep."

THE STONE

Lapis lazuli, or lazurite, is a deep blue stone with flecks of gold caused by iron pyrite and patches, or streaks of white caused by calcite. Good quality lapis is hard to find. Its name comes from the Persian word *lazward,* which means "blue." Ancient writers may have called it (and other blue stones) "sapphire." From early times it was prized and used for jewelry and ornaments. It is a stone that promotes fidelity and love. As you hold it in your hand and gaze upon its interesting features, it may impart to you a desire to seek out your mate.

THE GODDESS

On the face of it, Hera is the Greek goddess of marriage and Queen of all the gods and goddesses of Olympus. She was married to Zeus, the god of lightning and a major philanderer. The Greek myths present Hera as jealous, spiteful, full of rage and vengeance toward Zeus' many paramours (whether willing or not), and downright dangerous to the children from these unions. These dark aspects of the "goddess of marriage" hardly recommend Her as the agent and promoter of fidelity. However, we must understand that Hera's cult was older than that of the Olympians, and that She was the Great Mother Goddess in a matriarchal system long before She was relegated to the narrow patriarchal role of "wife." Her relationship with Zeus represented a battleground of sorts between one culture's attempts to overtake another.

Hera did retain Her triple aspect with the Greeks, as may be seen through Her titles: Hera Parthenos (maiden); Hera Telia (fully grown, complete); and Hera Chera (widowed or separated in some way from Her spouse). She also renewed Her virginity annually by bathing in a pool in Her homeland. This ritual represented a reclamation of self, symbolizing Hera's wholeness in and of Herself. By becoming complete in this way She is free to reconcile with Zeus as an equal.

This said, we may see that joy and deep love were also parts of Her relationship with Zeus. Their honeymoon after their *hieros gamos,* or sacred marriage, was said to have lasted for three hundred years. And though in Greek mythology Zeus treated Her abominably through His many dalliances, neither sought divorce from the other. The fact that Hera freely chose to work at salvaging their marriage, and was successful in Her own way, cuts through the darkness and finds that kernel of faithfulness that anchored Her deeply to Her wayward spouse.

This is not to say that if you are in a horrible, abnegating, and self-defeating relationship you should hang in there at all costs. Hera points to the need and desire for fidelity—of body, mind, heart, and soul—to be present in order for a relationship to have a chance to be forged between two separate people and their worlds.

Thus Hera may be invoked as Hera Telia, as Hera complete, in order to request Her to bless your union with the gift of fidelity.

THE MEDITATION (TO BE DONE IN CIRCLE)

You and your partner stand together in a natural glade. A pool of cool, clear water is before you; a waterfall spills into it from the heights. Luxuriant foliage grows all around. Peace and well-being fill you both. Clasping hands you walk together to a natural altar.

There you find two rings fitted with polished lapis lazuli stones, softly glowing. You stand together and call upon Hera, requesting Her blessing upon your union. She appears, rising from the pool in solitary splendor. She approaches the altar and smiles at you both. She holds Her hands out over the two rings, blessing and empowering them for the purpose of faithful union. The rings glow brightly in response. Hera instructs you to exchange rings. You gaze into each other's eyes and promise fidelity for as long as your union lasts.

Hera smiles and steps back into the pool. You and your partner kiss.

THE SPELL

Go to your ritual place. Set up your altar, cast your Circle, and request the presence of the Guardians. Invoke the goddess Hera, and in the presence of All, bless your stones by air, fire, water, earth, and spirit. Sit quietly before your altar and, with stones in hand, engage in the meditation. Keep your affirmation—that your bond of fidelity is passionate and deep—clearly before you. At the conclusion of the meditation, when it feels right to you, stand before your altar and intone the spell together, directing energy into your stones as you do so:

> Blue-eyed Hera
> exquisite queen,
> dignity and strength
> in Your every step,
> we call upon You
> and ask Your blessing
> upon our union.
> Bless us with the
> determination to be
> ever faithful—
> body, mind, heart, and spirit;

that we may live our love
with dignity and respect.
So mote it be.

When ready, give thanks to All present for Their assistance. Open the Circle and close the Temple.

You will want to wear your lapis lazuli rings as tokens of your promises and determination to remain faithful to one another. If infidelity by either partner should occur, that partner's ring may just decide to get lost.

THE TIMING

This spell is best done during new moon on either a Friday or Monday. Conduct the spell as dusk moves into night, ideally in a place where you can see the new crescent and the stars.

THE INCENSE

Lilac, rose, sweet pea, or myrrh.

THE CANDLES

Deep blue for fidelity, coupled with pink for love and red for passion.

THE PRACTICAL STEPS

- Simply doing this ritual with your mate will set up a resonance between you and an affirmation of the desire for fidelity.

- Set up a "love altar." Place upon it pink and red candles, cards you have given to each other, tokens of love. This altar is a living thing and you will remove and add things to it as your love unfolds. It will serve as a reminder of the love you have for each other.

- Open, honest communication should be a goal for both of you. Letting hurts fester or anger seethe are sure impairments to fidelity. Set up a regular time to meet and talk for the purpose of discussing anything that may be bothering you.

- Foster shared activities and interests. This will help you grow together rather than apart.

- Conversely, there needs to be time apart. Individuals occasionally have a need to be separate and alone. Solitude may be refreshing to some, so don't see this as a threat to your relationship.

- Appreciate and celebrate the differences between you. These differences are, in part, what attracted you to each other in the first place.

- If you have children, set up a time at least once a month for you and your mate to have a "date." This time is for the two of you to go out and have fun, and is not a time to discuss the children, jobs, in-laws, or the like!

THE PRIESTESS SPEAKS

To the acolyte bemoaning her fear that she will be unable to be faithful in her relationship to the Goddess and the God: "Every morning when you wake up, decide whether you will be faithful today. If the answer is 'yes,' the Gods will do the rest."

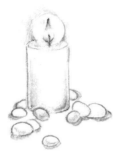

Tiamat: A Spell for Creative Chaos

THE MATERIALS

- Amazonite. This may be a natural unshaped stone, several polished beads, or other shapes.

- A pouch of bright green, the color of new leaves, made of soft but durable material. Or, if you will be wearing the beads, a cord for stringing them into a necklace or bracelet.

THE PURPOSE

The urge to create often begins in the dark, chaotic recesses of the soul. To create means to "bring into being from nothing" or "to cause to exist" (*Webster's New Twentieth Century Dictionary*, 427). This is a process. It may begin as a glimmer of thought, only to blossom into being as a poem, a painting, a garden, or anything else that calls forth effort from your deepest self. It is a force that often takes on a life of its own, and must be acknowledged in some form.

We all create in our own way. We write, paint, dance, plant, design, develop, teach, cook, sew, or make music. From the mundane to the sublime, every day may see us bring forth something new.

The satisfaction of creating, whether it is a meal to be shared among loved ones or a Pulitzer Prize winning story, is wholly for the self. It feeds the soul and opens the heart. Such satisfaction

73

ultimately allows us to be fully alive, and thus able to encompass others with our creative joy.

This spell is for the purpose of conjuring up creative energy. It is useful for helping you to embrace the chaos and lose yourself to the process, so something wholly new may be born.

THE AFFIRMATION

"I am a goddess (god) of creation."

THE STONE

Amazonite is a bright green or blue-green stone. It may be the color of new leaves. It can resemble some jades. Because of its color it is an excellent symbol of new beginnings. It is a stone of creativity, and according to author Judy Hall *(The Illustrated Guide to Crystals)* it is useful for wedding the intellect with intuition in order to fire the creative processes. Amazonite is lovely to look at, and engenders thoughts of newness and freshness, from which creativity may grow.

THE GODDESS

Tiamat is the Sumero-Babylonian Mother Goddess. From the chaos of formlessness She brought forth creation. She is affiliated with the waters of creation and is the personification of The Deep, or the eternal womb and the unconscious, from which life and creativity flow. She has been imaged as a great dragon or serpent. She is the raw material of creation, and thus is an appropriate goddess to summon when you wish to call forth your own creativity from the often-chaotic unconscious.

THE MEDITATION (TO BE DONE IN CIRCLE)

You are in a darkened space. There is no light, but you feel as if you are floating in warm water, and the gentle sound of lapping waves is very soothing. You have no fear. The darkness has a wait-ing quality to it. You hold your breath in anticipation. Then in the distance you see a light. It is a soft glow in the darkness. It comes closer, and as it does it illuminates where you are: a rounded cave. The water stirs, churning and heaving, yet you are still unafraid. Suddenly the light reveals a form in the darkness. A great serpent, green and gold, winged and crowned with flames. She rises from the waters and in Her claw She holds a glowing green amazonite stone. As you watch, She tosses the stone toward you, and within its heart you see a tiny storm of activity. You know instinctively that it is the key to your own creativity. The stone falls in the water before you, and without thinking you dive for it, following its soft green glow into the deeps. As your hand grasps it to yourself the water gives a great heave and you, with your prize, are poured from the darkness to the light. You know with certainty that you may tap into your creative self at any time, and find successful expression for your art, whatever it may be.

THE SPELL

Go to your ritual place. Set up your altar, cast your Circle, and request the presence of the Guardians. Invoke the goddess Tia-mat, and in the presence of All, bless your stone(s) by air, fire, water, earth, and spirit. Sit quietly before your altar and, with stone(s) in hand, engage in the meditation. Keep your affirma-tion—that you are a goddess (god) of creation—clearly before you. At the conclusion of the meditation, when it feels right to you, stand before your altar and intone the spell, directing energy into your stone(s) as you do so:

> Tiamat,
> great, heaving dragon
> of the night,
> of the deep,
> of the vast
> unknowable unconscious,

> reach into my
> chaotic thoughts
> and give them form.
> Release the creativity
> that is bound so that I,
> like You,
> may be the creator/creatrix
> of my world.
> So mote it be.

When ready, give thanks to All present for Their assistance. Open the Circle and close the Temple.

Since creativity may begin in darkness and chaos before emerging into the light of day and manifestation, keep your stone close to you, and ideally on your person, during any creative endeavor, even before beginning it. Sleep with the stone beneath your pillow so your creativity may be revealed in dreams.

THE TIMING

This spell is best done on a Wednesday. It should be done, if possible, on the night of the new moon, for you will be drawing chaos out of the darkness and transmuting it into creative energy.

THE INCENSE

Mint, fennel, lemon, peppermint, or any scent that tends to wake you up.

THE CANDLES

Yellow for stimulation coupled with light blue for creativity and red for passionate and positive activity.

THE PRACTICAL STEPS

- Sometimes we do not value our creative selves or we worry about what others will say about our efforts. Give some thought to your own attitudes and beliefs about creativity. Are they of value to you? If so, what makes them so? What barriers stand in the way of being creative? Do some of these beliefs and attitudes no longer hold true? Are there barriers of time or space that can be solved? Often before the creative energy can flow we need to understand what we feel and think about it.

- Set aside time and space for your creative endeavors. Commit some time each day to create. This will set up a habit of doing, until the energy can flow freely.

- If you've always wanted to paint, write, or cook gourmet meals but have no experience, join a class and just jump in. You won't know what you can do until you try.

- Join a group of writers, artists, jewelry makers, or whatever interests you. Having support as you go is good; you can learn from others and teach the newbies your art.

THE PRIESTESS SPEAKS

Upon walking into the acolyte's cell and seeing her whirling to the beat of drums, bright splotches of paint everywhere, and partially completed projects tossed hither and yon: "Er, I think you've got the chaos part down . . . ."

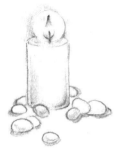

Whope: A Spell for Friendship

THE MATERIALS

- Turquoise, placed into a setting or upon a chain of silver either as a ring, earrings, necklace, bracelet, or anklet—even a belt buckle will do. You may need more than one, depending upon the number of people for whom you wish to invoke this spell.

THE PURPOSE

Friends. What would we do without them? They are the heart of our hearts. Unlike family members who may or may not be our friends, those we *choose* as friends are steadfast and ever at our side when needed. Friends are the people who listen to us uncritically, yet are willing to speak their truth to us. Friends are the ones we trust to keep the secrets of our hearts. They are the ones who commiserate with us over our woes, the ones with whom we share our joys, the ones who love us unconditionally, even when we are grumpy! Friends share our interests and activities, and are often the ones who may open new doors of opportunity for us.

In a true friendship there is always give and take. There is a balance in the ebb and flow of our lives. To have a friend, one must *be* a friend.

When we are children, it is easy to make friends. But often as we get older, the care and worries of our daily lives, the demands of our own families, and lack of opportunity make it difficulty to make friends. Treasure those you do have, and be sure to find time for each and every one.

It is interesting that so many television shows and movies are stories about friends. This contemporary interest in friends and friendships point to how important they are.

This spell is for the purpose of acknowledging our friends. It is a blessing upon our friendships, and a token of our esteem and hopes for long and fruitful relationships with those people we hold close to our hearts and call "friends."

THE AFFIRMATION

"To have a friend I will be a friend. I open my heart to my friends."

THE STONE

Turquoise is a stone that ranges in color from sky blue to blue-green to green. The stone has been prized for centuries and was used by the ancient Egyptians and Persians for jewelry and amulets. It was also known and used by the Aztecs and other people of South and Central America, but is probably better known because of its use by North American native peoples. For them it was prized by medicine men who used it for healing, to bring rain, and for protection. It has also long been a symbol of friendship and affection. Some say one should either give or receive it as a gift for the magic to work. It is an ideal stone to use to attract new friends to you, or to honor existing friendships.

THE GODDESS

Whope is a Lakota Sioux goddess. The Lakota were Great Plains people, living a nomadic life on the plains, hunting, fishing, and gathering the natural fruits of the earth. Whope is one of the most beautiful goddesses of this people. She represents peace, harmony, mediation, and the cycles of time. One of Her symbols is the peace pipe, which was said to be a gift from Her to Her people. Her name means *meteor,* and with each falling star she may grant a wish or mediate a problem between friends. This goddess, promoter of beauty and harmony, is perfect to call upon for blessing our friendships.

THE MEDITATION (TO BE DONE IN CIRCLE)

You find yourself on a vast plain. There is nothing but gently waving grasses for as far as the eye can see. The sky is blue, the color of a robin's egg. Wisps of milky clouds sweep its wide expanse. You turn and turn again and see a tepee rising against the sky. It is made of animal skins with brightly colored symbols decorating it. You are drawn to it. You enter, and there you see a beautiful maiden. She glows with spiritual energy and you know that She is a goddess. She gives you Her name: Whope. She is dressed in soft deer hides, decorated with exquisite beadwork and fringe. Her hair is black as a moonless night, Her eyes dark pools. Her skin radiates health and is the delicate color of sun-warmed terra cotta. She holds out a ring (or bracelet) to you of silver set with a beautiful turquoise. It seems to have captured a piece of the sky within it. You take it from Her and as you hold it in your cupped hands, She places Her hands over yours and utters a blessing upon it: "Harmony and peace between us through all the cycles of time." With that, you find yourself again upon the plain. But you are not alone, for you see your friend *(name)*. You go to your friend and place the ring into his or her hand. You then speak the blessing that Whope taught you: "Harmony and peace between us through all the cycles of time." Your friend receives your gift and accepts your blessing.

THE SPELL

Go to your ritual place. Set up your altar, cast your Circle, and request the presence of the Guardians. Invoke the goddess Whope, and in the presence of All, bless your stone(s) by air, fire, water, earth, and spirit. Sit quietly before your altar and, with stone(s) in hand, engage in the meditation. Keep your affirmation—that to have a friend you will be a friend, and will open your heart to your friends—clearly before you. At the conclusion of the meditation, when it feels right to you, stand before your altar and intone the spell, directing energy into your stone(s) as you do so:

> Talking grasses,
> whispering breeze,
> tumbling stars
> of eternity,
> Lakota goddess
> exalt this gift,
> and bless my friends
> through me.
> So mote it be.

When ready, give thanks to All present for their assistance. Open the Circle and close the Temple.

Plan on taking your friend or friends out for a meal and then present them with your gift. Explain that the turquoise signifies friendship and affection, and that you wish for beauty, harmony, and peace between you for all the cycles of time. If they accept the gift, they accept the blessing.

THE TIMING

This spell is best worked on a Friday, during the waxing moon.

THE INCENSE

Sweet grass or lemon grass.

THE CANDLES

Pink for friendship and love coupled with dark blue for understanding, patience, and peace.

THE PRACTICAL STEPS

- Write to a friend, but not by e-mail—send a good, old-fashioned card. This is a thoughtful gesture, showing that you have given time and thought to choosing just the right card for your friend. You might place some dried flowers, a pretty bookmark, or brightly colored confetti inside of the card.

- Call a friend you haven't spoken to in awhile. It is always good to hear a friendly voice.

- Invite a friend out to tea or brunch. Dress up for the event and make it special. Bring a little gift of a scented candle or a potted herb just to say "I love you."

- If you have just moved into a new area, get out and attend a local event. Volunteer at your library or children's school. Bake cookies for your closest neighbors and introduce yourself. It's sometimes hard to make new friends, but you can't do it without putting forth a little effort.

THE PRIESTESS SPEAKS

Noticing the acolyte hastily retreating from her office, the Priestess enters, only to find a small nosegay of herbs and blossoms left upon her desk. The Priestess smiles.

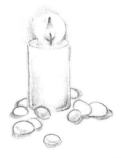

Pax: A Spell for Peace

THE MATERIALS

- Blue lace agate. This may be a natural, polished stone, or one or several stones fashioned into a piece of jewelry.

- A cord for stringing (if you will be wearing it), or another setting as desired.

THE PURPOSE

Peace. What does this word evoke? Is it a feeling within? Is it a quiet, restful environment? Is it a day without demands and disturbances in which you may do just what you want? Do you think of it in terms of only you, or does it encompass family, friends, and perhaps even the entire planet? *Webster's New Twentieth Century Dictionary* defines peace in many ways. They include: "calm; quiet; tranquility"; "to be or become silent and quiet"; and "freedom from war" (1317).

We all need to have times of calm. It is when we are at peace that our hearts may open. We may be more receptive to the realm of the spirit, and more inclined to share our peace with others, thus affecting our world in a positive way. It is while we are at peace that we may appreciate the gifts of the day, and embrace the night in untroubled slumber.

Often we are not aware of the importance of peace until it is gone, and then we may feel stressed and stretched, at odds with others and ourselves. Peace is necessary for the well-being of our minds and for the health of our bodies. Without it we cannot engage in the sort of quiet meditation that allows us to touch the face of Deity, from Whom all peace comes. This spell is for the purpose of engendering peace, within and without, for our good and the good of all.

THE AFFIRMATION

"I stand in the heart of peace. I share my peace with others."

THE STONE

The blue lace agate is one of my favorite stones. It is a delicate shade of blue, with subtle bands of white lace running throughout. It exudes peace, and when I hold it, I calm immediately. It may be used to invoke individual peace, or to affect an entire environment. It seldom fails to work its magic no matter how fractured one might feel. This is an excellent stone to use when peace of mind, body, or spirit is desired.

THE GODDESS

Pax is the Roman goddess of peace. The Pax Romana was the "Peace of Rome" known far and wide during the time of Rome's greatness. This goddess was depicted in white robes, holding an olive branch, cornucopia, and sheaf of grain, symbols of peace and plenty. In many church services the kiss of peace is given; thus, in spirit at least, this goddess is invoked. She may be called upon whenever you need peace in your life.

THE MEDITATION (TO BE DONE IN CIRCLE)

You find yourself standing upon the shores of a strange sea. The water is the color of azure and jade. The sky is rose and gold. A soft, fragrant breeze caresses your skin. You close your eyes and breathe deeply. Again . . . again. A sense of well-being and peace settles around you, within you. This magical place has touched your soul to its depths, and all is well. You smile. Opening your eyes you seek the horizon and you gasp in delight as you watch the earth rising. Higher and higher, a blue jewel, it rides the skies. It hangs there, too beautiful for words. As you watch, a soft light emanates from this gem and transforms before your eyes into a beautiful goddess. Her shining white robes drape elegantly around Her. She holds an olive branch in one hand; and a blue stone laced with white in the other. Her eyes are a soft blue, her hair golden, the color of ripe wheat. Her name is Pax, and She is a goddess of peace. She places Her hand upon your head and gives you Her blessing of peace. Offering you the stone, She tells you that, at need, it will impart a sense of peace to you and your surroundings. You accept the gift gratefully. She then places Her hands upon your shoulders and returns your attention to the earth. The internal peace that you feel reaches out with compassionate love to encompass this small miracle. The blue planet is laced in a white net of peace, just like your stone. Pax nods in approval and melts into the day. You bid farewell to these shores, and return home, holding peace ever in your heart.

THE SPELL

Go to your ritual place. Set up your altar, cast your Circle, and request the presence of the Guardians. Invoke the goddess Pax, and in the presence of All, bless your stone(s) by air, fire, water, earth, and spirit. Sit quietly before your altar and, with stone(s) in hand, engage in the meditation. Keep your affirmation—that you stand in the heart of peace and that you will share your peace with others—clearly before you. At the conclusion of the meditation, when it feels right to you, stand before your altar and intone the spell, directing energy into your stone(s) as you do so:

> Pax, bless me with Your peace . . .
> The peace of the Goddess is around me.
> The peace of the Goddess is above me.
> The peace of the Goddess is beneath me.
> The peace of the Goddess is within me.
> The peace of the Goddess flows through me.
> And I am blessed.
> So mote it be.

When ready, give thanks to All present for Their assistance. Open the Circle and close the Temple.

You may wear your blue lace agate daily as a reminder that peace is yours—and to remind you to *be* peaceful. When feeling a lack of peace, simply hold your stone and meditate the spell several times in conjunction with deep, relaxed breathing. You will feel a sense of peace and well-being after only a few repetitions. If you do not wear the stone, place it in a prominent place where you may see it daily: on your desk at work, in your car if you are prone to road rage, or in any spot where you can see it easily. If you handle the stone and repeat the spell regularly, you will feel more and more peaceful as you go about your daily activities.

THE TIMING

If you need peace between you and others, this spell is best done on a Sunday; if you seek inner peace, do this spell on a Monday. If possible, conduct this spell on the night of the full moon, with the moon's rays bathing you and your stone.

THE INCENSE

Any scent that makes you feel peaceful. Also consider gardenia, lavender, lilac, or violet.

THE CANDLES
Blue for peace.

THE PRACTICAL STEPS

- We may lose our sense of peace when we lose our sense of self. The Delphic Oracle's dictate to "Know thyself" is meaningful on so many levels. Knowing ourselves allows us to accept ourselves as we are, warts and all. It allows us to avoid the self-deceptions that can rob us of our peace. Knowing ourselves requires hard work and the ability to look deeply into the mirror of our souls. One way of doing this is to keep a journal. Keeping a journal is an excellent way of uncovering those self-defeating patterns that may rob or block our peace. Recognizing these patterns for what they are, we may take steps to do something to change them. It is, at least, a beginning.

- Two words: time management. This tool may be necessary if we have too many things going on. We may be like jugglers trying to keep too many balls in the air; some are going to hit the ground. Amidst all these demands and activities, there is no time to develop peace. Schedule the time you need to catch your breath. Take a bubble bath, a walk in the park, or share a special moment with a cherished friend. Then you may take this peace with you into your busy life.

- Make a list. Write down those things that fill you with peace, then resolve to do one thing at least every week.

- Take some time to meditate. Twice a day for twenty (even ten) minutes is all I ask! Go to your prayer place and sit before your altar, and simply let the Goddess and the God fill you with Their peace. Going to the source is one way of touching the vast reservoir of peace that is always available to you.

- Go to a peaceful environment—an arboretum, the beach, or out into the desert at dusk or dawn. Let the natural sounds of these places fill you. Nature has cycles of peace and tempest; from Her we may learn to have peace *within* the tempest.

THE PRIESTESS SPEAKS

The acolyte dashed hither and yon. Activity filled every waking moment and followed her into dreams. She did not notice what she lacked, but grew daily more irritable and grumpy. The Priestess, noticing this, stopped her in mid-run. She placed one hand upon her brow. "Peace be with you," she whispered. The acolyte felt a current of *something* pass through her. For that day, at least, she felt a sense of peace as she went about her tasks.

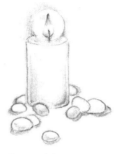

Vac: A Spell to Enhance Communication

THE MATERIALS

- Green aventurine. This may be either a single polished stone, or one or more stones fashioned into jewelry.

- A green pouch made of soft but durable material.

- Cord for stringing, if you will be making the stone(s) into jewelry.

THE PURPOSE

All beings communicate in some way. Humans do so with words in speech and writing. We send out signals by touch or look. Our body language may speak volumes, even when we are silent. Other creatures communicate by various sounds, behavior, and odors. Human babies communicate on a rudimentary level even at birth. Parents learn very quickly to distinguish cries of hunger from those a sick or angry child makes. Babies babble by the time they are two months old, mimicking those around them, and usually speak their first recognizable words—"mama" or "dada"—by around one year of age. As they master speech, they master their world.

Without communication we would be unable to make our wants and needs known; we may not even have the words for those things. We would not be able to interact with others, and society would be chaotic.

Communication, then, is vitally important. But we talk every day, don't we? And isn't that communication? How many wives have said to their husbands, "Are you listening?"; or how many parents have said to their teenagers, "Do you hear me?" Communication isn't just about talking, but listening and responding as well. It is giving thought before we speak.

Communication is an art, and one that many have never learned how to do successfully. In order to carry on a lasting love relationship or friendship, or to be competent parents, or to be successful in our work, we must know how to communicate appropriately and well. This spell is for the purpose of enhancing communication between you and loved ones, work colleagues, or in any situation in which communication is key.

THE AFFIRMATION

"Through the avenue of speech and the art of listening I communicate clearly."

THE STONE

Green aventurine is a stone embedded with flecks of fuchsite or hematite, and it may be transparent to opaque. It is often confused with green jade and may be sold as that stone. It is known as a good luck stone, and may be used to draw money to you. It is also said to balance the male and female energies and enhance the intellect. These latter traits make it an appropriate stone to use for communication—the heart and mind are balanced so the intellect may be clearly focused.

THE GODDESS

Vac is the Hindu goddess of the spoken word. She uttered the *Om* of creation, and presides over speech and oral communication. She imparts wisdom through incantations and mystic teaching. As a Mother goddess She is also concerned with creation. Since She spoke the first word and gave speech to Her people, She is an excellent goddess to call upon to help us with issues of communication. In Her creative aspect She may inspire the words She knows we hold in our hearts and set them free, like birds.

THE MEDITATION (TO BE DONE IN CIRCLE)

You find yourself in the midst of a great throng of people. All are talking at once, creating a cacophony of noise. You feel bewildered and utterly confused. You try to speak, but no words come forth. You utter a silent cry for quiet, for a time of respite between the many words. The scene begins to fade, as if overlaid with mist or a veil of delicate lace. From a Temple before you, a woman emerges and begins to walk toward you. She is too far away to be recognized, but wears a brightly colored silk sari that seems to float upon the breeze. As She grows closer you see that She has skin the color of coffee beans, and black hair partially covered by a gold cloth. Her face is lined and her eyes are ancient. She walks with dignity and grace. You try to greet Her, but no words pass your lips. Her eyes soften, and She reaches out and touches your throat, speaking the *Om* of creation. Suddenly words of thanksgiving burst forth from the recesses of your heart. The Goddess gives you Her Name: Vac. She takes you aside and teaches you about speech, then about listening and silence. She plucks a stone from Her hair and gives it to you as a reminder of your gift. The art of communication is yours and you may take your place among the throng, knowing this gift is always yours.

THE SPELL

Go to your ritual place. Set up your altar, cast your Circle, and request the presence of the Guardians. Invoke the goddess Vac, and in the presence of All, bless your stone(s) by air, fire, water, earth, and spirit. Sit quietly before your altar and, with stone(s) in hand, engage in the meditation. Keep your affirmation—that through speech and listening you communicate clearly—before you. At the conclusion of the meditation, when it feels right to you, stand before your altar and intone the spell, directing energy into your stone(s) as you do so:

> In the beginning
> was the word
> from which all
> creation sprang.
> My Lady Vac
> spoke and made it so.
> I call upon Her now
> for the gift of speech:
> with the clarity of rain;
> and the brightness of the sun;
> and the honesty of Her dark eyes.
> I shall speak,
> and like my Lady,
> make it so.
> So mote it be.

When ready, give thanks to All present for Their assistance. Open the Circle and close the Temple.

You may wear the aventurine whenever you will be facing situations where communication is important. The natural polished stone may be kept in a pocket or purse. When not in use, keep it in its green pouch.

THE TIMING

This spell is best worked on a Wednesday at the time of the new moon.

THE INCENSE

Anise, lemongrass, peppermint, or sage.

THE CANDLES

Yellow for communication. It may be combined with orange for action and stimulation.

THE PRACTICAL STEPS

- Sometimes speech does not come naturally or easily to us in certain situations. We may need to communicate in a meeting or before large groups of people, which can be a little scary. In order to overcome this public speaking anxiety it may be helpful to take a speech class. With repetition, speaking in front of others becomes easier.

- Join a club like Toastmasters. Such a group gives you a safe place to learn to be comfortable speaking before others about a variety of topics. They give guidance in communicating clearly and well. You might also have a lot of fun.

- Sometimes we do not speak what is in our hearts or heads because we are afraid, we don't know how to get our need or point across, or we feel unworthy. An assertiveness training class may help in these cases. Such classes help us to identify what we need to say and then teach us how to communicate it. With a little practice we may become better communicators, speaking our truths fearlessly.

- If you are shy about speaking out, it might help to practice what you want to say with a trusted friend, or you can even use that old standby—talking to your reflection in a mirror. Rehearse what you want to say over and over until you feel comfortable, then say it.

- Often we do not communicate well because we do not truly listen when the other person speaks. Practice giving your full attention to the other, rather than thinking about what you will say next.

- Take a creative writing class or a class in English composition if you feel you cannot communicate well through writing. Such classes offer us the tools, a chance to practice, and positive feedback on how we are doing. You might even discover you like the class!

THE PRIESTESS SPEAKS

The acolyte was brought before the Priestess for disciplinary action. While "experimenting" with herbs used for dying cloth, she turned everyone's undergarments woad blue! She was so busy coming up with an excuse that she was not listening as the Priestess spoke. Seeing this, the Priestess said, "The purple frog with pink stripes lives in your shoe," and was silent. The acolyte blurted out, "Yes, but I didn't know that woad, huh?" The Priestess said, "If you are going to speak, first be silent and listen. That includes quieting the mind and attending to the speaker."

Kupala: A Spell for Purification

THE MATERIALS

- Seven small aquamarines in their natural, unpolished state.

- Sea salt if possible, otherwise table salt will do.

- A small plastic bag in which to keep the salt, and a box in which to keep both the bag of salt and stones. You may paint the box a light blue or sea green, or decorate it with seashells if you wish.

THE PURPOSE

Many cultures and religions have purification rituals. During the Catholic Christian Mass the priest ritually purifies himself with water prior to offering the gifts of bread and wine. Men and women of Islam purify themselves before the five salats, or times of prayer, through ritual washing. Wiccans take a purification bath or shower using fragrant herbs prior to working magic or celebrating the Sabbats or Esbats.

There are particular times in religious practices to purify oneself in preparation for a closer union with the Divine. In Catholicism one must fast for one hour before receiving the Blessed Sacrament. The seasons of Advent and Lent are times of purification and meditation in celebration of the coming of the Lord, and in remembrance of His death and resurrection. In Islam the ninth month is called Ramadan, and is a time when people fast from food, water, rest, and sexual intercourse between the hours of sunrise and sunset in an effort to grow closer to Allah. In Wicca there are no special times or seasons of purification. However, a Wiccan may fast and meditate when there is a particular need in his or her life, or when he or she feels these methods of purification are called for. Whenever a Circle is cast the area is purified, and prior to worship within the Circle a Wiccan will take a purification bath or shower that usually utilizes salt and/or select rocks or minerals.

This spell is for the purpose of cleansing and purifying ourselves of those unwanted energies that hinder our communion with the Divine.

THE AFFIRMATION

"All negativity has left me. I am purified in thought, word, deed, and spirit."

THE STONE

Aquamarine comes in colors ranging from light blue to bluish green to pale sea green. It may look like a piece of frozen glacier ice. Its name means "sea water," from the Latin *aqua* (water) and *mare* (sea). It has long been associated with the sea and with water deities, and has been used for both protection and purification.

Salt is a mineral associated with the earth. It has been prized through the ages for a variety of reasons. It lends flavor and zest to foods, and was used as a preservative, thus ensuring against famine during harsh winters when food was scarce. It can also be used for destruction by sowing fields with it, rendering the fields sterile, unable to support life. Salt was, and is, used in religious rituals. Traditionally in Catholicism, salt was added to water while blessing it as an act of purification. It was placed on babies' tongues during baptism to call forth wisdom and preserve the child from the devil's wiles. In Buddhism, salt, water, and fire have been used for purposes of purification. In Wicca, salt has always been used for purification and protection. Blessed salt may be added to charged water, which is then sprinkled around the area in which a Circle will be cast. Salt and water may be used for blessing and purifying the home or ritual articles.

Together, aquamarine and salt are excellent minerals to use for the purposes of purification and cleansing.

THE GODDESS

Kupala is the Slavonic water goddess associated with springs and rivers. Her worshippers bathed themselves while calling on Her name in order to purify themselves. They also collected dew on the night of Her festival to use for the same purpose. Water is a powerful element of purification, as it absorbs and neutralizes negative energy and lets it simply wash away. Kupala also has a fire aspect. Fire is often used for purification, burning off the dross to get at the gold within. She is an excellent goddess to call on for any purification rite.

THE MEDITATION (TO BE DONE IN CIRCLE)

You find yourself in a glade. Lush green ferns and evergreens surround you. In the center is a spring that bubbles up from the depths of the earth. You hear its music, giving cadence to the songs of birds and the hypnotic drone of insects. The sky is a delicate blue, and the breeze is scented with pine and warm stones. You are wearing a soft gray robe that feels like mist or spider's silk. You let it slip off, to pool around your feet as you enter the spring. You find that the water is cool but not cold. Refreshing. You sink beneath the surface and allow your thoughts to become one with the water. As you seek the surface you call upon Kupala, Lady of this spring, to wash away all hurts and negativity. She rises from the water in concert with you. Her hair is the delicate color of water lilies and flows out behind her like a living thing. Her skin is milky. Her eyes, the color of blue ice, look into your soul. She comes to you, this half wild spirit, and with cupped hands full of water baptizes you in the name of Goddess, in the name of God. Through Her blessing you are cleansed and purified of all unwanted energies. She reaches beneath the water and draws forth seven stones, the color of Her eyes. These She holds out to you, an external sign of your inner purification. She then places a pinch of salt upon your tongue, a preservative against the return of the unwanted negativity. You exit the spring and collect your robe, bidding farewell to Kupala as She sinks beneath the waters.

THE SPELL

Go to your ritual place. Set up your altar, cast your Circle, and request the presence of the Guardians. Invoke the goddess Kupala, and in the presence of All, bless your stones by air, fire, water, earth, and spirit. Sit quietly before your altar and, with stones in hand, engage in the meditation. Keep your affirmation—that all negativity has left you and you are purified in thought, word, deed, and spirit—clearly before you. At the conclusion of the meditation, when it feels right to you, stand before your altar and intone the spell, directing energy into your stone as you do so:

> Kupala, Lady of the stream,
> with water, salt, and aquamarine,
> cleanse me—body, heart, and soul,
> that I may arise complete and whole.
> Release me from all negative thought
> that sin and sadness come to naught.
> And bless me with Your cleansing grace,
> and preserve the memory of Thine embrace.
> So mote it be.

When ready, give thanks to All present for Their assistance. Open the Circle and close the Temple.

Keep the salt and stones in your box upon your altar, if you have one. If ever you need purification or a cleansing blessing, take them out, then do the meditation and speak the spell.

THE TIMING

This spell should be worked on a Saturday, when the sun is at its zenith, to take advantage of the fire aspect of Kupala. It should be worked during the waning moon, as we are essentially binding or banishing negativity from our lives.

THE INCENSE

Camphor or eucalyptus.

THE CANDLES

Black candles to absorb and release all negative energies, and white candles as a symbol of purification. Light both at the beginning of your meditation. At the conclusion of invoking Kupala and intoning the spell, allow the candles to continue burning until they are completely burned down. Be sure they are kept in a safe place.

THE PRACTICAL STEPS

- Take a purification bath in order to release all negativity from your body. This will help relieve the stress and tension we often hold in our bodies. Run a bath at a temperature that is comfortable for you. Sprinkle some of the charged salt in the water, as well as any oils or bubble bath that you like. Light black and white candles, and place your aquamarines either in the bath or around the candles. Have some soft music playing in the background. As you soak in the water, repeat Kupala's spell. All stress and tension will fade away.

- Bless and purify your home with the house blessing ritual in the appendix, or create your own ritual. Use your charged salt, and place the aquamarines in the water bowl.

- Meditate in order to clear your mind and purify your thoughts. Do the chakra meditation found in part five, "Divination with Stones," in order to align and cleanse your psychic centers.

- Place some charged salt and aquamarines around your home or office to transform negative energies into positive ones.

THE PRIESTESS SPEAKS

The acolyte watched in awe as the Priestess gracefully entered the sacred spring where she intoned a spell for purification. The moon shone bright and full. The energies thrummed all around them. The acolyte, imitating her mentor, approached the spring with regal bearing, where she promptly slipped and fell, face forward, hitting the water with a mighty splash! The Priestess, hair dripping around her face, held her hand out to the wayward girl and said, "I think you may dispense with the spell; you most assuredly have the Goddess' attention."

Artemis: A Spell for Autonomy

THE MATERIALS

- One splendid tiger-eye. This may be a loose polished stone, or a stone set in a ring or pendent.

THE PURPOSE

Autonomy is the gift of self-governance. With such a gift comes great responsibility. It is a freedom within limits, and with great latitude for doing good or evil. It is not for the weak of heart to seek, for it sometimes demands that one walks a solitary path. Sacrifice is part of its nature, as is compassion.

An autonomous person is one who ultimately walks alone. One who has a set of personal ethics that is unbendable and always for the greater good. Often such a person will stand in opposition to the majority, and may be the one to point out a truth others are unwilling to see. Strength and courage are necessary attributes for an autonomous person. He or she must set ego needs aside (the need to please and to be liked), and must always seek to live a genuine, congruent life.

This spell is to help anyone on the path toward autonomy, toward that genuine life where all our parts create a whole in conjunction with the Divine.

THE AFFIRMATION

"Do what thou wilt shall be the whole of the Law. Love under law, love under will" (*Book of the Law,* 9).

THE STONE

Tiger-eye is a variety of quartz. It is opaque and has bands of brown, from yellow-brown to almost black. As the stone is turned in the light, the dark bands become lighter and the lighter become darker. It is a lovely, mysterious stone, constantly changing. Tiger-eye may be used to develop confidence and independence, to become attuned to your inner resources and strengths, and to promote personal responsibility. Just as it seems to change but remains its essential self, so too may a person grow and change, but always hold fast to his or her moral and ethical convictions. This stone is excellent to use in a spell for autonomy, because all of its properties are necessary for that state of being.

THE GODDESS

Artemis was born of Leto with Zeus as Her father, though She may have ties to earlier cultures as a Great Mother Goddess. At an early age Artemis requested of Her father that She be allowed perpetual virginity and to be given the mountains and wild places for Her home. She rejected the normal roles for women of the time, becoming completely autonomous, her own woman. She was Protectress of the wilderness and the animals there, and took special care of young girls and women. She was midwife to laboring women and guided the newborn into this life. As nurturer She was known as the Many-Breasted Artemis at Her shrine in Ephesus, where She was a threat to the burgeoning Christian sect.

Artemis lived freely. She lived by a set of moral and ethical standards that were unbreakable, and those who trespassed against them—and Her—were shown justice without mercy. Though a Protectress of animals, She was also the Huntress, running under the full moon with Her hounds where She took those sick and weak animals, or those needed only for food and clothing. Her physical prowess and grace are a part of Her persona, a symbol of Her freedom.

Somewhat contradictory—solitary yet seeking the company of Her nymphs; Protectress and Huntress by turns—Artemis is a good role model for those of you who need to find and set limits, both for yourself or for what you will allow in your life. She may guide you toward finding what is needed in order to live an authentic life. Artemis is the ideal goddess to call upon when seeking autonomy, though She may be demanding and exacting should you choose to follow Her path.

THE MEDITATION (TO BE DONE IN CIRCLE)

You awaken in a mountain fastness. You arise, alert and aware. You are wearing a chiton, a short, white garment, yet you revel in the coolness of the morning. Before you is a crude altar upon which is a statue of Artemis, holding a bow, surrounded by Her hounds, a hart leaping before Her. A stone flashes in the rising sun, first bright, then dark, flecks of gold catching fire as the light plays over the stone. It reminds you of the juxtaposition of light and dark, day and night, life and death. You reach out to touch it. Instantly, the hart takes flight, hounds leaping after her, and Artemis stands before you. You stand and gaze at each other, face-to-face, Her in Her glory, you in strength and courage. The remoteness in Her eyes retreats, giving way to tawny warmth. She recognizes you as a fellow journeyer of the wild places, those places in the heart and mind of those who would follow Her. She casually picks up the blinking, knowing tiger-eye—Her token of acceptance—from the altar and tosses it to you. By receiving the stone you promise to walk the path joyfully, with strength, courage, and determination, with full responsibility for your acts, with compassionate justice, and with your integrity before you like a shield. No one may rule over you unless you abdicate your goddess-given power. You take up the blessing and the challenge, and follow Artemis into the woods.

THE SPELL

Go to your ritual place. Set up your altar, cast your Circle, and request the presence of the Guardians. Invoke the goddess Artemis, and in the presence of All, bless your stone by air, fire, water, earth, and spirit. Sit quietly before your altar and, with stone in hand, engage in the meditation. Keep your affirmation—that you may do what you will so long as the guiding hand of love is present—clearly before you. At the conclusion of the meditation, when it feels right to you, stand before your altar and intone the spell, directing energy into your stone as you do so:

> I am born of the wind.
> I live in the flame.
> The waters of life sustain me.
> The rich fertile earth upholds me.
> I glide through the heart of the forest
> unseen except as a reflection of the moon.
> I am one with the creatures there;
> my hair grows like meadowsweet.
> I am She who Is,
> untouched, unattainable, eternal,
> like the stars hidden beneath the mask of the day,
> or like the Huntress
> swift and terrible.
> So mote it be.

When ready, give thanks to All present for Their assistance. Open the Circle and close the Temple.

Keep the tiger-eye upon your person, either in a pocket or worn as jewelry. It is your cloak of autonomy and a reminder that you are She who Is.

THE TIMING

This spell is best worked on a Sunday or Tuesday just after the new moon. Repeat the spell every Sunday until the moon is full.

THE INCENSE

Pine, frankincense, or sandalwood.

THE CANDLES

Red for strength, courage, and passion coupled with gray for wisdom and dark blue for self-awareness.

THE PRACTICAL STEPS

- In order to be autonomous one must have a sense of self. In order to do this one must know what one stands for and believes in. Try this exercise: take a piece of paper and write on the top "I believe in . . . ," then list those beliefs you hold dear. Some examples are "I believe in being honest" or "I believe in always being nice." This list should also include some of the hard beliefs such as those you hold about abortion, welfare and "the poor," religion, and so on. Then take each of these beliefs and reflect on how they play out in your life. If there are any inconsistencies, take a closer look at them to determine why. Perhaps a belief you have held dear is not really yours, but someone else's. Or perhaps you are not the person you once were. You should give time and thought to this exercise. It can be done over a period of days or weeks.

- Courage is necessary to live autonomously. Courage stems from the heart. Men and women in the armed services who show unusual courage are awarded the Purple Heart as a symbol of that courage. We may say "My heart quailed" when faced with a frightening situation. Take some time and meditate on what courage means to you. See how you may live more courageously each day, perhaps by speaking up if you see some wrongdoing, or refraining from gossip or even putting a stop to it. There are many opportunities throughout each day for acts of courage, and even small acts of courage may lead to great changes.

- Think about what you have chosen for your life, and what you continue to choose. Take personal responsibility for those choices. Do not hide the fact of your decisions from yourself, but claim them. If they are not right for you, change them.

- Take time to seek the solitary places. Go to the beach, the mountains, or even your own backyard. Allow yourself to appreciate your surroundings and connect with the natural world. See your place therein and claim it.

- Become active in a sport. It does not have to be strenuous or too demanding: a brisk daily walk, badminton, tennis, tai chi, yoga—whatever will get the blood moving. Revel in your body, in the way it works during these activities, and enjoy how you feel afterward.

THE PRIESTESS SPEAKS

The acolyte, wearing a white chiton, left breast bare, took bow and arrow and, with exquisite concentration, hit the bull's eye of her target. With fluid grace and beauty she drew another arrow, again placing it where she wanted it. Seemingly unseen, she danced in pure joy at her accomplishment. The Priestess, watching in her scrying bowl, smiled, seeing the woman the acolyte was on her way to becoming.

Sophia: A Spell to Increase Wisdom

THE MATERIALS

- Two labradorite stones. They may be worked into a piece of jewelry or left as natural, polished stones.

- A pouch made of soft but durable material in which to keep the stones when not in use. It may be a soft shade of gray or the blue of a tropical butterfly's wings. A fabric that has an iridescent sheen would be ideal.

THE PURPOSE

Ah the folly of youth! Those uncounted days of exploration and revelry; a time when action was often not connected to thought, and when we thought we would live forever and that the world would open to us like a cracked egg, spilling its golden contents into our hands; a time when all too often, like the Fool of the tarot, we trod close to the cliff's edge in blissful ignorance with never a care in the world.

Folly, like a raging, tumbling stream, is primitive and untamed. Wisdom takes that wild stream and fashions it into the deeps of a clear mountain lake or the fathomless sea. Folly blazes the trail that Wisdom transforms into a path, open to all but traveled by few. Wisdom is the stillness that Folly swirls around in chaotic disarray, seeking that still center.

Wisdom comes from experience, knowledge, inner insights and discernment. Young children often display wisdom, before they are molded into societal patterns that dampen their natural knowing. Wisdom is not necessarily related to age, but we are more willing to accept that only the Elders may be wise. Conversely, in our modern, technological society we may view elders as useless and as a drain of resources. Wisdom often stands in opposition to what is popular. Wisdom seeks to lead us into realms of thought that open us to Divinity. The wise person is never harsh and condemning of individuals, only of those practices or patterns of thought that keep people slaves to themselves, to others, or to ideas of oppression. Wisdom may fling open the shutters of the stale house of our soul, letting in light and life and unlimited possibilities.

This spell is for the purpose of increasing Wisdom in our lives. Wisdom is not only a desired quality, it is a living force. We may recognize Her if we are willing.

THE AFFIRMATION

"I embrace Wisdom, and invite Her into my heart, mind, and soul."

THE STONE

Labradorite is a plagioclass feldspar. It is an unassuming gray stone, until one takes a closer look. Then, as the light touches it, it seems to catch fire all along its surface, revealing patches of iridescent blue the color of a tropical butterfly's wings, or the scales of a fish reflected in the sunlight. This phenomenon coined the term "labradorescence." It is so startling to see, it evokes a smile and sets one's thoughts spiraling to images of mystery and revelation. It has been used to raise consciousness and increase insight. By meditating on this stone one may come to that Divine Mind that leads to Wisdom. It is an appropriate stone to use in order to increase the awareness of Wisdom's presence in one's life.

THE GODDESS

Sophia is the Gnostic Goddess of Wisdom. It was She who generated the cosmos out of Herself. She was the first light within the
darkness and gives the gift of gnosis or knowing to women and
men. As Wisdom She was also mentioned in Hebrew writings and
was said to have danced before the throne of God before the
world began. In the *Book of Wisdom* much is said about Her:
"Resplendent and unfading is Wisdom, and she is readily per-
ceived by those who love her" (*New American Bible,* 780), and elsewhere, the wise ". . . shall shine brightly like the splendor of the
firmament" (ibid., 1060). Wisdom was highly praised, and many
positive and desirable attributes were ascribed to Her. Eastern
Christians also revered Sophia, and the best known shrine to Her
is the church of Hagia Sophia, or Holy Wisdom. In the Jewish
Qabalah Wisdom resides in the second sephirah, Chokmah.

Though attempts were made to de-deify Her, She continued to
be part of the cult and culture of the early monotheistic religions
and survives even today in one of Mary's titles: Throne (or Seat)
of Wisdom. Sophia is a good goddess to call upon to lead you in
the path of Wisdom.

THE MEDITATION (TO BE DONE IN CIRCLE)

A Priestess meets you at the Temple's gates. She is dressed all in
white and can hardly be seen due to the light she gives off. You,
too, are clad only in white, with a wreath of lavender upon your
brow. The Priestess leads you through the gates and into the Temple, where you find yourself before the Throne of Wisdom. Seated
upon the Throne is an unprepossessing woman. Her robes shimmer in the lamplight, not any one color but reflecting all colors.
Two pillars stand on either side of Her; at first sight they are gray,
but as the light plays over them they seem to flash with an inner
fire, reminiscent of the inside of an abalone shell. The pillar on
the left is named Silence; the one on the right, Knowing. The
goddess Sophia, for that is who She is, waves you forward. You

climb up three steps and stand before Her. She places the palm of Her right hand upon your brow; Her left hand is raised before your lips, indicating silence. For it is in silence that Wisdom may fly to you, gifting you with the knowing that you need. Your eyes flutter closed, and when you come to your senses you find yourself outside of the Temple gates. But in your hands you find two stones, fashioned of the material of the two great pillars. You know that Wisdom will always be with you—if you are but wise enough to heed Her.

THE SPELL

Go to your ritual place. Set up your altar, cast your Circle, and request the presence of the Guardians. Invoke the goddess Sophia, and in the presence of All, bless your stones by air, fire, water, earth, and spirit. Sit quietly before your altar and, with stones in hand, engage in the meditation. Keep your affirmation—that you embrace Wisdom and invite Her into your heart, mind, and soul—clearly before you. At the conclusion of the meditation, when it feels right to you, stand before your altar and intone the spell, directing energy into your stones as you do so:

> Throne of Wisdom,
> Shining Countenance,
> You who danced at the
> foundations of the world,
> I seek to know,
> to will, to dare, and
> to keep silent,
> a Priestess of the Wise.
> Grant that when I speak,
> I do so with intelligence and knowledge;
> when I will,
> I do so with pure intention;
> when I act,

I do so with integrity;
and in silence
may I open to the Divine Mind.
So mote it be.

When ready, give thanks to All present for Their gracious assistance. Open the Circle and close the Temple.

You may wear the stones or keep them close to you in situations where wisdom is particularly important. When not in use they should remain in their pouch.

THE TIMING

This spell is best worked on a Wednesday or a Saturday at the time of the full moon.

THE INCENSE

Almond, anise, or sage.

THE CANDLES

Dark blue for wisdom and self-awareness coupled with purple for opening oneself to the Divine Mind.

THE PRACTICAL STEPS

- Be silent. Quiet your inner self through meditation. Quiet your outer self by thinking before you speak, and speaking only that which is necessary and efficacious to others. All too often we chatter, both inwardly and outwardly. Be silent and let Divine Wisdom guide your thoughts and words.

- View all who come your way as teachers. We may learn from others, including animals, plants, stones, and spirit-friends. All have wisdom to share, so remain open and ready to receive that wisdom.

- Be a teacher to others. Share your knowledge. As you teach, so also do you learn in greater depth.

- Practice some form of divination. By opening yourself to the Divine Mind and tapping into your own intuitive self, Wisdom may make Herself available to you.

THE PRIESTESS SPEAKS

The acolyte was busy chattering to her newer sisters, showing off her wisdom and knowledge. Her poor sisters were becoming confused and overwhelmed. The Priestess, noticing this, called the acolyte to her side. Still chattering and not really paying attention, the acolyte bumped squarely into the Priestess. The Priestess looked deeply into the acolyte's eyes and simply raised her left hand to her lips, indicating silence. Immediately the acolyte was stuck dumb, but at the same moment she was also struck with a realization: the beginning of wisdom was the realization that she didn't know everything, and that everything she knew wasn't necessarily wise. It was in silence that she would be able to hear Wisdom sing and find discernment in the song.

Lakshmi: A Spell for Abundance

THE MATERIALS

- Four small, natural, cut and polished peridot stones.

THE PURPOSE

Abundance is having more than enough. More of what? It may be money and wealth, or food to eat and shelter for the body. It may be a loving family and caring friends, or robust health. Abundance may also be spiritual in nature, an overwhelming connection with the Divine. However it is defined, abundance is more far-reaching than simple prosperity, and encompasses the entirety of one's life.

We all desire abundance; we do not consciously seek out want. The tricky thing about abundance, however, is that we must recognize it when we have it. It is all too easy to want more, better, bigger, and costlier. Keeping up with or being one step ahead of the neighbors isn't abundance. Rather, it is a sad attempt to shore up one's fragile ego, to "find" happiness in material possessions, to build confidence by pointing out the number of toys one has acquired. But this is the path to disappointment and debt, and it has nothing to do with abundance.

Two things are necessary for abundance. The first is the willingness to receive: we must remain open, willing, and ready to receive abundance. The second is gratitude: we must allow ourselves to feel thankful for what we receive, and recognize the gifts we are all too often given without asking.

One may have abundance in the midst of poverty, or live in lack of it as a millionaire. Abundance is having more than enough, and if we are honest with ourselves, most of us receive this gift every day. This spell is for the purpose of helping us recognize the abundance we have in our lives, and when there is a lack, to attract that which will fill the need.

THE AFFIRMATION

"I have abundance in all the facets of my life."

THE STONE

Peridot, also called olivine, is a transparent green stone. Traditionally olivine is more olive-green in color, while peridot is a clear spring green. Peridot tends to be used as a precious stone in jewelry. Its lovely clear green color tends to make one think of new growth and new beginnings. It is a springtime stone, and has the energy and drive of that season. It has traditionally been used for luck, prosperity, and money spells, so it is appropriate to use for calling abundance into your life.

THE GODDESS

Lakshmi is a Hindu goddess who represents wealth, prosperity, good fortune, harvest, and abundance. In addition, She is the active female principle, or Shakti, in the male deity. She was also the giver of sovereignty and a model of devotion to Her spouse, Vishnu. She is a very benign goddess, and wishes to share Her wealth with those who approach Her. Her energy is that of a mother giving to Her children, thus She is an ideal goddess to call upon when abundance is needed.

THE MEDITATION (TO BE DONE IN CIRCLE)

You find yourself within the atrium of a stone Temple. You sense that it is of a great age, yet the floors have a high polish to them and the bas relief carvings look newly completed. Plants grow lushly from large colorful pots. Vines have begun their trek around huge pillars. A water fountain plays its music at the center. You begin to walk toward a pair of giant doors made of polished brass with intricate carvings all over them. You are dressed in a lovely sari of green and gold that flows soundlessly as you move. As you approach the doors, they open of themselves, a soft perfume wafting out to envelop you. As you enter this light-filled room you see the goddess Lakshmi upon a dais toward the front. She sits serenely in the lotus position, actually floating in the air. Beneath Her are lotus flowers of many colors, all in full bloom. To either side of Her are fountains fashioned to look like elephants. Their trunks reach out and send a fine spray of water onto the flowers. Golden light emanates from this goddess and a clear green peridot rests in the center of Her brow, glowing softly. Her hands stretch out gracefully toward you as Her eyes open, mirroring the stone upon Her forehead. From Her hands all manner of goodness falls—health, money, bountiful harvest, palaces, and love. All are yours to take; abundance is within your reach, which you accept with gratitude and praise. The Goddess places into your hands four small peridots, seeds for future abundance. With these riches you bow and leave Her presence.

THE SPELL

Go to your ritual place. Set up your altar, cast your Circle, and request the presence of the Guardians. Invoke the goddess Lakshmi, and in the presence of All, bless your stones by air, fire, water, earth, and spirit. Sit quietly before your altar and, with stones in hand, engage in the meditation. Keep your affirmation—that you have abundance in all the facets of your life—clearly before you. At the conclusion of the meditation, when it feels right to you, stand before your altar and intone the spell, directing energy into your stones as you do so:

> Lakshmi, Golden One,
> giver of all gifts,
> Patroness of Abundance,
> give to me that which
> I need for my sufficiency.
> Whether health, or
> the land's bounty,
> loving family and friends,
> shelter, or the means of support,
> grant me a boon from
> Your substance.
> With gratitude and thanks
> I accept Your gifts.
> So mote it be.

When ready, give thanks to All present for Their gracious assistance. Open the Circle and close the Temple.

The peridots may be used for any area of your life where you need abundance. For example, one may be placed with your bank or other financial account papers, or one may be carried with you for abundance of positive feelings and interactions throughout your day. If you need a home you may place one wrapped within a picture representing the type of home you desire, then place that on your altar; or one may be placed in your kitchen to represent abundance of physical sustenance.

You may invoke the spell frequently, charging your stones on a regular basis.

THE TIMING

This spell should be worked on a Thursday after the new moon.

THE INCENSE
Allspice, cedar, ginger, or sassafras.

THE CANDLES
Green, the color of new growth. The green candles may be coupled with yellow, for attraction.

THE PRACTICAL STEPS
- Too often we do not feel we "deserve" abundance. Get over it! Be open, willing, and ready to receive. See yourself as deserving of Lakshmi's gifts. If your sense of not being good enough or not deserving the good things in life cannot be overcome, it might be helpful to seek out a counselor so you can get to the root of this false belief.

- When you wake up in the morning give thanks for the bounty you have in your life: your family, friends, pets, home, and other possessions, the ability to support yourself, good health—anything for which you are grateful. Before you go to sleep at night consider all the bounty you have received throughout the day. Gratitude is an important and necessary component of abundance.

- Give cheerfully! Find a religious institution or charity, such as your local animal shelter, and give a portion of what has been given to you. Give of your time by volunteering to help a child or an adult learn to read at your local library, or collect food for the local food bank. These are ways of passing your abundance on to others. The more you give, the more you will have.

- Remember, abundance is often a state of mind.

- For money matters, open up a savings account or begin an investment portfolio. You do not need to be rich to do either, simply commit a portion of each paycheck to them, or similar endeavors. If you feel you do not know enough about investing, go to your local library and check out some books, or seek the advice of an investment counselor.

- Get rid of all but one credit card, and call this your "emergency" card. Define "emergency" clearly! Credit card debt is one of the things that people fall into and often find it difficult to get out of. If you can, go by the motto "If I can't pay cash, I don't need it."

- Work on defining "need" and "want." Abundance will fulfill our needs, plus give us a little left over for our wants. Just don't get the two mixed up!

THE PRIESTESS SPEAKS

The Priestess entered the acolyte's cell. She saw a bewildering array of things: books piled into towers ready to topple, bowls full of fruit and candy, empty soda cans, clothes strewn all about . . . more things than she could count. She felt her temper begin to flare and went in search of the greedy girl. She found her in the Temple, placing fresh flowers before a statue of the goddess of plenty. Bowing, the acolyte gave thanks for all of the abundance in her life. The Priestess silently withdrew, understanding that the acolyte, though perhaps a bit messy in her abundance, had a grasp of gratitude and was able to express it.

Athena: A Spell for Success in the World

THE MATERIALS

- Four carnelian stones bound together. They may be worn as jewelry, or simply kept together in a pouch.

- A pouch made of soft but durable material the color of the stones you select.

THE PURPOSE

While on this earth most of us must live in the world. We have certain worldly pursuits that enable us to be independent and responsible people. Most of us work for our living. By possessing a job or career we earn money to purchase those things we need and want, but more importantly, if we're lucky, we follow the vocation of our hearts. Doing what we like gives us intangible rewards such as a sense of wholeness, success, confidence, self-satisfaction, joy—all things that money can't buy. I view success in the world as living a congruent life where doing and being are in perfect harmony.

How many of us spend our time at jobs that drag at the heart and deaden the soul? How often do we go to work in silent despair, knowing it's what we *have* to do in order to make ends meet? We actually spend the majority of our waking time working, and may spend more time with our colleagues than with our own families. If this is the case, isn't it important that the time we spend in these pursuits and with these people be well spent?

It often takes time and many false starts to find our place in the world. That's why, at forty-something, I am still trying to figure out what I want to be when I grow up! View these false starts as part of the learning experience and then move on, knowing you were doing what you needed to do at the time. Eventually you will find your niche, and when you do you'll be eager to do the work and will receive joy, as well as a paycheck, for your time.

This spell is for the person who desires success in the world. It will help you find your way to that particular vocation that will enhance, rather than detract from, your life.

THE AFFIRMATION

"I experience success as I joyously embrace my life's work."

THE STONE

Carnelian may range in color from pink to orange to reddish-orange. Traditionally it has had many uses and has been assigned many attributes. It aids in finding one's life path and making positive choices. It helps in planning and organizing, as well as manifesting one's plans. It may impart energy and dispel apathy, increasing concentration and follow through. It has been used for career success and positive connections with new opportunities. As such, it is an excellent stone to use for success in the world.

THE GODDESS

Athena is Her Father's daughter. One of Her myths states that She was born fully-grown and armed out of the split skull of Her Father Zeus after He swallowed Metis ("Wisdom"), Her Mother. Athena identified with the status quo and some would say She was a cop-out to the patriarchal culture of the time. However, according to Her most popular legends, She was ever-virgin (a woman unto Herself) and determined Her own path in life. She was resourceful, resilient, intelligent, articulate, self-disciplined, an excellent strategist, ruler, and protector of the city of Athens who moved comfortably in the then male-dominated world. She was a born leader and counseled the heroes of the times. She was an inventor and creator, said to have taught crafts such as weaving and spinning, and to open men's minds to literature, art, law, and judgment. One of Her symbols is the olive tree, which signifies peace, victory, and abundance. Her sacred animal is the owl, representing wisdom, no doubt, and She has some relationship to serpents. The serpent may represent a connection to an older version of the Goddess as Great Mother Goddess, and survived upon Athena's shield in the form of the snake-headed Medusa.

Athena is an ideal goddess to call upon for success in the world, for that is Her realm.

THE MEDITATION (TO BE DONE IN CIRCLE)

Prior to this meditation, sit quietly and let your mind open to the many vocations that are available to you. Ignore any barriers, such as education requirements, salary needs, or past work experience. Simply look at these possibilities and choose one thing that you think you would like to do. Then begin.

You find yourself in your ideal job setting, be it in a high rise on Wall Street, a dairy farm in the Midwest, a computer center in Silicon Valley, and so on. You are dressed for the part. Imagine the sounds, sights, and smells that you would experience there. Watch your colleagues as they go about their work. Take some time to get a feel for what it is like to *be* what you have chosen to be. As you become comfortable with this role, you see striding toward you an authoritative-looking woman. She is dressed perfectly for the setting, Her dark brown hair is pulled back into a stylish

chignon, Her gray eyes are alive with intelligence, and Her hand-
shake is firm. She takes you under Her wing and shows you
around, and She shows supreme confidence in your ability to do
the job. You feel alive, excited, full of interest and curiosity. You
feel an energy that feeds you, and you just *know* that you have
found your right place in the world of work. This modern Athena
at your side is completely at home here. Before She leaves you to
your work, She hands you four glowing stones, a reminder that
anything is possible. Now it is time for you to begin.

THE SPELL

Go to your ritual place. Set up your altar, cast your Circle, and
request the presence of the Guardians. Invoke the goddess
Athena, and in the presence of All, bless your stones by air, fire,
water, earth, and spirit. Sit quietly before your altar and, with
stones in hand, engage in the meditation. Keep your affirmation—that you experience success as you joyfully embrace your
life's work—clearly before you. At the conclusion of the meditation, when it feels right to you, stand before your altar and intone
the spell, directing energy into your stones as you do so:

> The opportunities of the heart
> are all arrayed before me.
> Athena leads the way;
> I have only to choose.
> I seek the path that leads
> to success, to inner satisfaction
> and confidence.
> I seek the path that fills
> my days with joy and celebration.
> For who I am, and what I do,
> symbolize inner harmony
> and ultimately reveals the
> contentment of the soul.
> So mote it be.

When ready, give thanks to All present for Their gracious assistance. Open the Circle and close the Temple.

The carnelians should be kept together and either worn as you seek your right vocation or kept in their pouch under your pillow, where dreams may be a clue to your path. They may also be kept upon your altar, as a daily reminder to meditate upon your need.

THE TIMING

This spell is best worked on a Thursday after the new moon.

THE INCENSE

Anise, hyacinth, or rosemary.

THE CANDLES

Yellow for action and drawing desired results to you; orange for communication and stimulation; and green for financial prosperity.

THE PRACTICAL STEPS

- If you are already in a job you like but the spark has seemed to go out of it, take some time to stand back and evaluate it—and your needs. Write out a list of the things that energize you about your job, the things that are a drag, and something you would like to see done differently. Then take a look at the list and see how you can work more of the things you like to do into your day; see what changes you can make regarding the things you don't like; and how you can insert a new idea or program you are excited about into your work. Often a job that has gone "dry" just needs a new approach.

- If you are unhappy with your job, go to the library and check out some of the many books concerning careers and career changes, and begin to explore the careers that are available and the steps it would take to make a change.

- Engage the services of a career counselor. These counselors are trained to help you find what you like to do, and will help you get started.

- Check out offerings at your local night school or college. If you're not sure what you want to do, take some classes in subjects that are of interest to you. Sometimes by doing this you have an "ah-ha" experience and discover just what you want to be when you grow up!

- Volunteer, if possible, at a place where you may be interested in working. Often by working in the environment you get a sense of whether or not it's for you.

- If you are drawn to certain jobs, interview different people who work in those fields. Talking with people who actually do the work is often helpful.

- Pay attention to what you do for "fun." Sometimes these activities may be turned into a paying proposition. Also pay attention to dreams, including daydreams, which offer clues to your interests.

THE PRIESTESS SPEAKS

The acolyte, like a lovely butterfly, flitted from job to job within Goddess House. Nothing seemed to fit and she was becoming discouraged. The Priestess asked her one day, after all of her soufflés fell during a turn in the kitchen, what she *liked* to do. The acolyte promptly responded, "I like to read." The next day the Priestess apprenticed the acolyte to the Mistress of the Books in the library, where she happily settled in. All agreed that she was a wonderful library assistant.

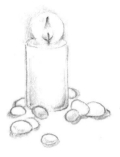

Maat: A Spell for Justice

THE MATERIALS

- One piece of jade. It may be used in a necklace or a ring, or may be in the form of a single jade bangle bracelet. It may be a piece that is carved into the likeness of a feather, or left as a natural polished stone.

THE PURPOSE

Justice without mercy is vengeance. I think about the day the United States suffered a concerted terrorist attack resulting in tremendous loss of life, property, and the sense of personal and national security. When I heard about and later viewed the effects of the attacks I was filled with grief, fear, and a growing desire for vengeance. I had to work hard to check this latter feeling and to turn it into a thirst for justice instead. Justice without mercy is vengeance. We are a people of justice, and must continue to shine in the darkness of loss, fear, and anger to be a light to the rest of the world.

Justice presupposes a sense of fairness and impartiality that allows the truth of a matter to be revealed. The job of justice is to present this truth so that a matter may be judged and resolved for the higher good. One must set aside one's personal beliefs, prejudices, or desires in order to be fair so that the truth may be honored.

This spell is for the purpose of invoking justice in your life in a personal, or even national, matter.

THE AFFIRMATION

"In the interest of justice I am blind to all but the truth."

THE STONE

Jade is a stone that was known and loved by the ancients. There are actually two types of jade: jadeite and nephrite. Jadeite is harder than nephrite, though both were used in carvings and for jewelry. We commonly think of jade as being a rich green in color, but it can also be pale green, white, black, pink, and yellow. Jade has been carved into images of the Chinese goddess Kuan Yin and the Buddha. It also has a connection to Maat, the Egyptian goddess of justice. Jade may be used when justice is desired, and to lend positive energy to uncover the truth of a matter. It may be used to shed light on court cases and legal disputes. It is a good choice for drawing justice into your life, and to remind you to act in a just manner toward all.

THE GODDESS

Maat, or Mayet, is the Egyptian goddess of justice and truth. She stands for the cosmic order and replaced chaos, being the Light that Ra, Her Father, brought to the world from out of the darkness. Her symbol is the ostrich feather, and when people die, their hearts are weighed against this upon Maat's scales. If the heart is free of evil and balances with the feather of truth, the soul is conducted to the throne of Osiris, god of the underworld, and thus welcomed into the afterlife. But if it fails in the balance, the monster Ammut, who is part lion and part crocodile, devours the soul. The Pharoahs of Egypt ruled only under Her consent, and no one, not even the other gods and goddesses, was above Her. As goddess of the divine order all must be judged against Her justice at some time. As goddess of balance, She is also concerned with maintaining the balance of our lives in all that we do. Maat is an excellent goddess to invoke when justice and truth are needed; when light is needed to shine upon the darkness of ignorance and evil.

THE MEDITATION (TO BE DONE IN CIRCLE)

You stand within the Halls of Justice before a statue of Maat, who is holding the feather of Truth. Her robed priests and priestesses are arrayed before Her. They wear black, and cowls hide their faces. Pillars stand to the right and left of Her, one black and one white. Scales, balanced and waiting, are at Her right hand; the sword of justice and of vengeance is poised to Her left. Your heart quakes within you; how will you be judged? A bell sounds, sweet and clear. Incense clouds the air. Maat opens Her eyes, no longer a lifeless statue but the goddess in all Her power. Her green eyes bore into you, reading your very soul. Slowly She places the feather of truth upon the scales and takes up the sword. As you watch, the scales tip, then balance; you have been judged and you pass the test. The sword is placed at rest. A priestess comes forward and robes you in black. The Goddess gives you a jade piece, a symbol of your new position as defender of justice. You go forth from Her presence, knowing in your heart that you are changed from this moment on. You will be a proponent of truth, the Goddess' agent in the world.

THE SPELL

Go to your ritual place. Set up your altar, cast your Circle, and request the presence of the Guardians. Invoke the goddess Maat, and in the presence of All, bless your stone by air, fire, water, earth, and spirit. Sit quietly before your altar and, with stone in hand, engage in the meditation. Keep your affirmation—that in the interest of justice you are blind to all but the truth—clearly before you. At the conclusion of the meditation, when it feels right to you, stand before your altar and intone the spell, directing energy into your stone as you do so:

> Clear-eyed agent
> of justice
> You are blind to all
> but truth.
> Fairness covers You;
> You hold the scales
> that weigh the heart
> in balance
> with serene impartiality.
> To You do I advocate
> my cause;
> from You will I receive
> Your just reply.
> Maat, settle upon me
> Your feather of truth.
> So mote it be.

When ready, give thanks to All present for Their gracious assistance. Open the Circle and close the Temple.

Wear or carry your jade piece as a reminder that you are an agent of Maat's justice in the world, and to draw needed justice to your cause.

THE TIMING

This spell is best worked on a Thursday in the full light of day at noon. The mid-point between the new and full moon is recommended. It may also be worked on the equinoxes, times of balance.

THE INCENSE

Sandalwood.

THE CANDLES

White for pure intentions and black for binding or releasing, in this case, injustice.

THE PRACTICAL STEPS

- Seeking for the truth in the name of justice requires that you set aside your biases and be aware of your prejudices. Take some time to explore these for yourself, especially about the important issues such as abortion, race relations, religion, politics, and the like. It is useful to be aware of where we stand on various issues, and how they may affect our search for truth and justice.

- When in a dispute or when mediating one, now that you know what your biases and prejudices are, *listen* to the other side, remaining as neutral as you can. You may not change your stance or decision, but your decision will be with the full knowledge of what drives you. Justice implies fairness and impartiality. Strive for these attitudes when justice is needed.

- Join a group that works on larger issues of justice. It may be something like Amnesty International or, considering justice for the planet, Greenpeace. There may be an organization in your city that helps battered women or abused children. Your involvement might just tip the scales so that justice may be served.

- Meditate upon your life and your relationships with family, friends, and colleagues. Are justice and truth present, or do you need to make some changes to let them in? If we cannot live a just life with those closest to us, we will never be able to do so in the wider world.

THE PRIESTESS SPEAKS

The Priestess stands at the altar within the circle of standing stones. She holds before her a sword. It is double edged. One edge represents justice, the other vengeance. Around her are her priestesses, each holding candles, black and white. A terrible injustice has come to the land. The acolyte approaches the Priestess, white feather of truth held tightly in her sweating hand. With a cry the Priestess raises the sword and sweeps it down, to stop trembling at the tip of the feather. Vengeance, confronted by truth, is turned aside. Mercy becomes the guiding hand and justice will prevail.

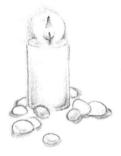

Persephone: A Spell for Transformation

THE MATERIALS

- A single opal that holds shifting light and fire within its heart. It should be worn in a piece of jewelry.

THE PURPOSE

Like the butterfly who must retreat into the silence, solitude, and darkness of its cocoon before emerging in radiant beauty, we too often go through our own process of transformation at different points of our lives. When we leave home for the first time, finish college, get married, have a child, or take leave of someone we love, we go through a process of change and become someone different than who we were. We are forever changed. Sometimes these changes are happy ones, but others are full of sorrow. Those times when it seems that we lose all sense of direction, when hope fades or despair encroaches upon us, are the very times that offer the greatest opportunities for growth and change. It is in the darkness that the seed first germinates; it is in the silence and solitude of our soul's truth that we learn to become who we are meant to be.

Transformation is a process of becoming. Like the snake who sheds her skin to allow for new growth, we too shed old manners of living and being in order to resonate more fully with our life's purpose and with the Deity who first breathed life into our souls. We discover that loss is an illusion and learn that the real riches are those that cannot be captured or cataloged.

Some of us voluntarily retreat from the world's commotion in order to take stock of our lives and determine if we are living a life in harmony with what it takes to reach our full potential. We must shed the caterpillar's skin and flex our wings, often leaping into the unknown with the faith that the winds of transformation will uphold us.

THE AFFIRMATION

"I embrace my process of becoming, knowing that loss is but the gateway to growth."

THE STONE

The opal was known to the ancients as a good luck stone, but somewhere along the way it got the reputation for causing bad luck. It is never used in engagement rings for this reason. Opal is a stone that contains water molecules within it, thus this stone should not be left near heat, nor should it be cleansed by placing it in direct sunlight, as this could cause it to become dull. Fluctuating temperatures may also cause it to fracture. These warnings aside, it is a beautiful stone and comes in a variety of colors, including milky-white, yellow, brownish-yellow, brown, brick red to hyacinth red, green, mossy green, black, clear, and the popular variegated type that flashes with inner fire. Besides being a good luck stone, it may be used in astral projection, psychic practices, connecting with higher realms, and inducing visions. Gazing into this multicolored stone that shines with an inner fire, one can well imagine that it will open the gates of the unconscious and be a light in the darkness of becoming. This stone is my choice when invoking or embracing one's transformative processes.

THE GODDESS

Persephone is the darker self of the Kore, Maiden of sweetness, light, and innocence. She is the mature Woman who has come into power only after a transformative experience. She has found liberation through and within the darkness, though for Her, this process was frightening and terrible. Yet she took those experiences and fashioned for Herself an entire realm. As queen of the underworld, of the unconscious, and of death, She has experienced enlightenment and is an appropriate guide for others who find themselves in the darkness.

Transformation may also begin in the light. As Kore She enjoyed the sunshine and beautiful wildflowers, the impossibly blue sky, and the companionship of Her friends. She never realized, until the moment was upon Her, that She would be utterly and irrevocably changed.

Whether our particular transformations are products of the darkness or the light, Persephone is an excellent goddess to be our guide, to bring us to the center of our souls.

THE MEDITATION (TO BE DONE IN CIRCLE)

You find yourself in a dark tunnel. There is warmth, and not too far away you hear the sound of trickling water. From the corner of your eye you glimpse a presence, all in black. She (for you sense that it is a woman) moves away from you, deeper into the earth. Lacking any other ideas of what to do, you follow. The tunnel winds 'round and 'round, deeper and deeper toward a center as yet unseen. As you follow the downward spiral it becomes warmer and warmer, and as you go you leave your clothing behind, until all you are wearing is a filmy loincloth. Your breasts glisten with perspiration, you hair lies in damp curls down your back. Finally you come to a halt. You find yourself in a large round chamber, richly appointed. The draperies are in shades of lush purple and glittering black, the floor is polished obsidian. A thousand candles in silver holders light the room. In the center of the room is a large fire pit, embers glowing green, then red, then blue; colors the opulent hues of gemstones and starlight. The veiled Woman stands before the pit and motions you forward. Hesitantly you approach. The goddess of this underworld, Persephone, throws back Her veil and studies you with eyes of jet. She reaches into the dancing, multicolored flames and draws forth a perfect opal. It has captured the flames within its heart. Silently, She hands it to you, then stands away from the pit. You understand what you are to do. Clutching the gem, you leap without thought into the flames and for a blinding instant of ecstasy all possibilities are open to you, even death. You spread wings you never knew you had and take flight upon the warm air currents, rising until you reach the chamber's heights and break through to the light. Gently you come to earth, the joy of transformation, like twin stars, shining from your eyes.

THE SPELL

Go to your ritual place. Set up your altar, cast your Circle, and request the presence of the Guardians. Invoke the goddess Persephone, and in the presence of All, bless your stone by air, fire, water, earth, and spirit. Sit quietly before your altar and, with stone in hand, engage in the meditation. Keep your affirmation—that you embrace your process of becoming, knowing that loss is but a gateway to growth—clearly before you. At the conclusion of the meditation, when it feels right to you, stand before your altar and intone the spell, directing energy into your stone as you do so.

> Lifting from the confines
> of earth,
> tremulous wings unfurled,
> nature's colors in flight,
> my spirit breaks free
> and soars.

> Emerging from the tenebrous dark,
> wind blowing away the
> clinging shadows,
> I enter into the light
> surfacing into ecstasy.
> Persephone,
> goddess of the night,
> wrap me
> within Thine ebon cloak as
> I seek the death of
> becoming.
> So mote it be.

When ready, give thanks to All present for Their gracious assistance. Open the Circle and close the Temple.

You should wear your opal while sleeping so your unconscious may release its transformative powers. During the day it may be worn as a reminder that change is in the air whenever Goddess is in our lives.

THE TIMING

Transformation often begins in the dark. If possible, work this spell on a Saturday while the moon Herself is dark, just before She becomes a sliver of new light in the night sky. Midnight is a good time, when all is still.

THE INCENSE

Frankincense.

THE CANDLES

Gold, a reminder that we must pass through the flames of transformation before our new, true self may shine through.

THE PRACTICAL STEPS

- Keep a dream journal in order to become aware of your inner processes and patterns. Place a notebook and pen by your bed and as soon as you awaken capture the images on paper lest they fade away with the coming of the sun. Meditate on the images and see what comes up for you. Buy a dream dictionary to see what the images and symbols might mean, but don't rely on it, as your inner truth may speak louder than someone else's definitions.

- Meditate regularly. This will help you to get in touch with your center and allow unconscious thought to rise to conscious awareness, and it will allow you to connect with the Divine Mind.

- Engage in stream-of-consciousness journaling, or get out the crayons, finger-paints, or other art materials and let your imagination flow. These activities may reveal your transformative process.

- Drum. Let the pounding rhythms of the drums, a language all their own, speak to you. When it feels right, stop. Then jot down the thoughts and feelings that come to mind.

- Be open to all possibilities!

THE PRIESTESS SPEAKS

Concerned about the acolyte's growing silence and quiet withdrawal from the community, the Priestess dipped into her dreams. There she saw bright flittering butterflies and iridescent dragon scales; brilliant snakes shedding gossamer skins and pools of liquid colors, merging and flowing in bright swirls. . . . The Priestess quietly withdrew, recognizing the acolyte's transformative process.

Madame Pele: A Spell for Protection

THE MATERIALS

- Several small pieces of lava rock.

- Sea salt.

- A small box, painted red and decorated as you wish, in which to keep the salt.

THE PURPOSE

Within our mothers' wombs we are protected and secure. Sometimes I think we unconsciously spend much of our lives seeking that sense of security again. The world is often harsh and can be a scary place in which to try and make one's way. On some level we remember how we felt while floating gently in the warmth of our mothers' bodies, and long for that feeling again.

The need for protection encompasses many aspects of our lives. Personal protection, and protection for our possessions, our home, and our good name are all important to us. We desire protection for our children and those we love from the vagaries of life and ill health or ill luck. We strongly protect our feelings from those we feel we cannot trust, and just as strongly share them with those we can trust.

When one is protected one feels safe. A sense of security allows one to *breathe* and to pursue those things that are important to us: love, careers, material possessions, creative pursuits, creating a family, and seeking knowledge. Feeling protected frees up energy for these things, and though feeling protected is often a state of mind, practical steps may be taken to both physically and psychically promote protection. This spell will draw a mantle of protection around you and give you an ally during times of strife.

THE AFFIRMATION

"I am safe and protected at all times."

THE STONES

Lava is a product of volcanic activity. It is produced through the combined activity of fire and earth, and air and water. Thus it contains the four elements. It is also infused with spirit, as it represents both dark and light, destruction and construction, and death and life. The stone is receptive and can absorb negative energies from the environment. Because of this it may be used in any protection spell.

Salt is a mineral associated with the earth. It was, and is, used in religious rituals. Besides its use for the purification of objects, people, and sacred spaces, it is also an excellent mineral to use for protection. A Circle of salt will keep psychic attack or entities at bay. Sprinkling blessed salt around your home will act as a repellent to any negativity. A packet of salt may be carried with you for the same purpose.

Used together, salt and lava are excellent to use in a spell for protection.

THE GODDESS

Madame Pele is said to have come from Tahiti to Hawaii by canoe. Once there, She proceeded to create all of the landmasses of

Hawaii through volcanic activity in order to create a home for Herself and the growing numbers of Her worshippers. She is still actively acknowledged, if not worshiped, in that island state. She appears either as a very old woman, or a younger one dressed all in red dancing on the rim of a volcano. Her temper is fiery, and She can release the hidden fires within Her mountains for destructive purposes if She is riled. But in the end, even Her acts of destruction allow for new growth in the dark rich soil formed from the molten rocks and ash. She is so protective of Her home that people who take away souvenirs of it without first asking are beset with bad luck, and for this reason careless tourists send rocks and pieces of lava back to Hawaii every year! Pele is a good goddess to call upon for protection. Just be sure you offer a gift as a thank you. Suitable ones include cigarettes (tobacco), coins, strawberries, flowers, and any strong alcoholic drinks.

THE MEDITATION (TO BE DONE IN CIRCLE)

You find yourself upon the side of a mountain. It is bleak, ashy, barren. The scent of sulfur assaults you, and heat curls around your feet. You wonder what you are doing here. You move forward on a barely discernable path to reach the summit. Upon the rim you stand, buffeted by hot clouds of air. Spread out before you is an inverted cone, red embers against glassy black rock. You are standing at the edge of a volcano's maw, and you can see a pool of molten lava heaving beneath your feet. Strangely, you feel no fear, only a growing curiosity. As you watch the glowing panorama before you, it seems to part. Rising from the depths is a goddess, for who else could possibly survive in this place? She is dressed all in red and has black hair and eyes that glitter like obsidian. She comes to stand before you. Her skin seems to glow with inner heat. She welcomes you to Her home, and with a motion of Her hand, opens out before you a shining vista. You see Her mantle of protection flowing out from Her shoulders to cover the land. Though fiery of temper, Her first duty is to protect what is Hers. You have a sense of peace and security knowing that Pele is watching out for you. As a reminder of Her security and as a bond for it Pele gifts you with pieces of Her mountain home, lava rocks that hold a memory of the earth's fire. You return home, cherishing this gift of Pele's heart.

THE SPELL

Go to your ritual place. Set up your altar, cast your Circle, and request the presence of the Guardians. Invoke the goddess Pele, and in the presence of All, bless your stones by air, fire, water, earth, and spirit. Sit quietly before your altar and, with stones in hand, engage in the meditation. Keep your affirmation—that you are always safe and protected—clearly before you. At the conclusion of the meditation, when it feels right to you, stand before your altar and intone the spell, directing energy into your stones as you do so:

> Pele's fire,
> a molten flow,
> to use for destruction
> or help new life grow.
> She lives in the earth's depths
> so far below,
> but stirs in anger
> at sight of a foe.
> Pele's fire,
> a gentle flame,
> peace and protection
> are yours to attain.
> By calling upon Her,
> by saying Her name,
> fears without and within
> you'll be able to tame.
> So mote it be.

When ready, give thanks to All present for Their assistance. Open the Circle and Close the Temple.

Be sure to offer the fire goddess a gift in thanks. Set out a bowl of strawberries; crumble a cigarette into the fire or the earth; toss some coins over your left shoulder; pour strong spirits onto the earth (never in the fire!); or make a lei of flowers to set upon your altar. Pele will bless you for it.

Scatter the lava rocks before your front door, symbolically setting up a barrier to negative energy. Sprinkle the salt around the inside of your home or place some in a small bowl to set upon your altar. Put some in a small bag to put in your car or carry with you for protection away from home. Renew the salt periodically and keep it in your box in case of need.

THE TIMING

This spell is best worked on a Sunday at around noon, when the fire of the sun is at its most fierce. It should be during a time of the moon's waxing.

THE INCENSE

Allspice, hyssop, or tobacco.

THE CANDLES

White for protection; and red for the goddess Pele, for strength, and for passion.

THE PRACTICAL STEPS

- Practice the meditation regularly until you can bring Pele's protection to you at a thought. Being filled with a sense of inner confidence about your personal safety will alleviate many anxieties.

- Take reasonable precautions for your home, personal possessions, and car. Make sure locks are good, and use them. If you wish, install alarms in home and car. Take out insurance against loss, in case the worst does happen. These activities may add to your peace of mind.

- Hone your awareness of what goes on around you by becoming *aware*. Do not place yourself in questionable situations. Don't become a victim.

- Take a self-defense class and practice the moves regularly. Don't hesitate to protect yourself when you need to.

- Start a Neighborhood Watch. Get to know your neighbors. They are the ones who will watch out for your home when you're not around.

- Ward your home against psychic incursions. Use the house-blessing ritual in the appendix.

- Don't let your fears get the better of you. If you are unreasonably afraid all the time, seek counseling.

THE PRIESTESS SPEAKS

The acolyte was anxiously setting wards around her cell. She was very conscious of her personal safety because prior to coming to Goddess House she had suffered from some unfortunate experiences. Her anxiety sometimes kept her from sleeping. The Priestess, noticing this, went to the acolyte's cell and spoke with her soothingly. She then gave her a token, charged with her own personal energy, for the acolyte to keep with her always. The acolyte gratefully placed it in the pocket of her robe, releasing a long pent-up sigh. The Priestess quietly left, knowing that with the sense of psychological safety, the acolyte would sleep well tonight.

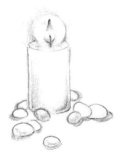

The Moirae: A Spell to Accept the Cycles of Our Lives

THE MATERIALS

- A single piece of petrified wood, large enough to appreciate the various bands of color and shapes most contain.

THE PURPOSE

A tree reveals the cycles of its life when, through accident or design, it is brought down, leaving behind nothing but a stump. But the stump contains the entire history, not only of the tree, but also of the surrounding environment. By counting the rings it is possible to determine the age of the tree. By studying the rings one may ascertain the climatic conditions of each year: was rainfall plentiful or was there a drought? Were conditions right to allow this or that disease or pest to attack the tree? Did the tree have all of the nutrients necessary to thrive? When a tree falls in the forest with no one to see, does it still sing its death cry to the universe, and was its life of value simply through its being?

There are cycles of the moon, the tides, the seasons, and our lives. We are born, live out our span for good and ill, and die. Some say there was a beginning before our beginning, and no ending when we die. Some see life in a linear pattern: from here to there, then gone. Others see life as a spiral (a shape so prevalent in nature) and view each year we live as adding to the never-ending cycle of our being, like prayer beads upon a string.

Each cycle teaches us something, if we are but willing to learn. And as we grow from babe, to toddler, to child, to adolescent, to young adult, to middle age, to elder, and finally go to meet our death, we must accept the passages that each age offers. It does no good to go kicking and screaming into that good night, nor is there reason to.

Each cycle of days is a gift. Each one is an irretrievable gem. We grow, we learn, we make mistakes, we love, we lose, we hurt, we triumph; we experience life to its fullest in all its guises. The thread of life shows bright and dark but ever adds to the tapestry of existence. When we pass beyond this world we might see the entirety of the work, but upon this earthly plain we are far too concerned with our own little thread to be able to see the whole.

This spell is for anyone who desires to accept the cycles of his or her life, to embrace the passages from one stage to another, and to anticipate the changes that come to us all. It may be worked at any time when we feel a shift, a change, or catch a realization that we are passing from one phase to the next in our lives.

THE AFFIRMATION

"I cycle around from life to death to life again in perfect acceptance."

THE STONE

Petrified wood began life as a living tree. When it died, minerals replaced the organic material and it became fossilized; the tree turned to stone. Petrified wood is beautiful to look at and invites one to touch and hold it. I have a piece I have had over thirty years; it is a link to my distant past! This wood-turned-rock is a reminder of the cycles of change and the new forms that may grow out of them. It is a good symbol of the uncounted cycles of our lives, and so it is appropriate to use for this spell.

THE GODDESS

The Moirae are actually three goddesses, the Greek Fates. The first is Clotho, the Spinner. She spins the threads of our lives, her distaff ever turning like a top. The second is Lachesis, the Measurer. She measures out the threads of our lives and (I like to think) is also the Weaver who creates great beauty out of them. The third goddess is Atropos, the Cutter or the Inevitable One, for She is the goddess who cuts the threads of our lives and finishes the pattern. These goddesses cannot be denied. They are ever the bringers of change, and unfold the cycles of our lives with grace and imperturbability. They are excellent goddesses to call upon for accepting the cycles of one's life.

THE MEDITATION (TO BE DONE IN CIRCLE)

You find yourself in a hut. It is made of stone and has a dirt floor and a thatched roof. It is clean and neat, well-lit by a cheerful fire in the large hearth. You feel comfortable and warm. You realize that you are not alone. There are three old women off to one side of the hearth, the fire casting them alternately in light and shadow. They do not seem to notice you, as They are busily engaged in Their own activities. One is spinning bunches of soft wool into fine thread; the second is measuring out the thread and using it to weave with, but you cannot make out the pattern; the third is standing by holding wicked-looking shears, occasionally sniping a thread the Weaver holds out to Her. Their movements, along with the flickering fire, mesmerize you, and you take a step closer to Them. Immediately They stop what They are doing and fix bright, birdlike eyes upon you. "Come here, dear," says the first one. "I am Clotho, and I spin the thread of your life." "To Me," says the second. "I am Lachesis, and I weave your thread into the whole of existence." "And I am Atropos," says the third. "When the time is ordained, I snip the thread and send you on your way to Another's hands." You blink and take a step backward. Together, the three say, "Changes and changes are yours to know. Cycles within cycles are yours to grow. We spin, We weave, We cut the thread. Living and dying are nothing to dread." Then They all make a shooing motion with Their hands and you find yourself outside of the hut. As a reminder of your visit you pick up a rock from the garden. It has patterns within it and changing colors, and is very, very old. It was once a living tree, but through time and change is now a conglomerate of living minerals. It is an appropriate reminder of the changes of life and the goddesses who ordain them.

THE SPELL

Go to your ritual place. Set up your altar, cast your Circle, and request the presence of the Guardians. Invoke the goddesses Clotho, Lachesis, and Atropos, and in the presence of All, bless your stone by air, fire, water, earth, and spirit. Sit quietly before your altar and, with stone in hand, engage in the meditation. Keep your affirmation—that you cycle around from life to death and life again with perfect acceptance—clearly before you. At the conclusion of the meditation, when it feels right to you, stand before your altar and intone the spell, directing energy into your stone as you do so:

> Spinning, whirling,
> twisting, twirling,
> Clotho spins the
> thread of life.
> Assessing, plaiting,
> measuring, merging,
> Lachesis weaves the
> strand of life.

> Dissolving, breaking,
> disbanding, parting,
> Atropos cuts the
> cord of life.
> Changes within changes
> are mine to know.
> Cycles within cycles
> are mine to grow.
> You spin, You weave,
> You cut the thread.
> I know that
> living and dying
> are nothing to dread.
> So mote it be.

When ready, give thanks to All present for Their assistance. Open the Circle and Close the Temple.

Keep the piece of petrified wood on your altar, or anywhere that you will see it regularly. It is a reminder of the cycles of your life, and the wonderful changes that await you at every step. As you approach a particular change you may hold the stone and meditate upon it, receiving clarity and strength as you do so.

THE TIMING

This spell should be worked on a Monday. It may be worked during any phase of the moon, depending upon the cycle you are leaving or entering. For example, the dark of the moon could be for contemplating death and for preparing for it, or it could be for gestating change and preparing for new beginnings. The full moon could be a completion of one phase prior to letting it go and releasing that which is no longer needed or desired in your life. Meditate upon the cycle, change, or passage you are in or about to experience, and then decide where it fits in the moon's cycle.

THE INCENSE
Sandalwood.

THE CANDLES
White for the moon and Her cycles, and dark blue for change. Other colors may be added or used, depending on what cycle or passage you are celebrating.

THE PRACTICAL STEPS

- We cannot accept what we do not understand. Understanding the tapestry of our lives is never an easy thing to do. This exercise is to help you "get a handle" on your life. You are going to create your personal history (or "herstory") from birth to the present time. You may do so by writing your own autobiography; you may draw and paint those significant points in your life; you may do a timeline. Be sure to note your ages at the various points. Make it as detailed as you can. This can take a period of days or even weeks.

- Now that you have your personal history, identify recurring themes or cycles. Note the significant passages you have experienced. What are they? In what ways do they keep recurring, if they do? How do you feel about them? At what ages do these cycles recur? What meaning do you ascribe to them? Who are you in these situations? This study will allow you to attend to incomplete cycles or even identify destructive cycles. Once known they may be changed.

- Document your experiences during a chosen cycle: a day, a week, from one full moon to the next, or throughout the Wheel of the Year. What changes do you notice during this time? What lessons are you gifted with?

- If you are struggling with a passage in your life it helps to be able to talk with others who are going through the same thing.

Look around for a support group you can join and share the struggle, drawing strength.

- Create a ritual you can do alone or with others to celebrate the changes in your life. A ritual engages one psychologically, emotionally, and physically, and can be great fun as well!

- Keep a Book of Changes documenting the significant events in your life. Include pictures, thoughts, feelings, souvenirs, and so on. It may be a bittersweet experience to look through it, but nevertheless, it is the story of your life.

- If coping with a difficult passages, seek counseling in order to gain perspective and support. Like giving birth, moving into a new stage of life may be difficult, and you may need a midwife.

THE PRIESTESS SPEAKS

The acolyte lovingly placed the stuffed animals and dolls of her youth into a box and placed it outside of her cell, to be donated to a local shelter. She felt it was time to put away these childish things, for wasn't she on the sacred path to serving Goddess? The Priestess happened by a little later, and noticed the box sitting there. At the end of a long day the acolyte returned to her cell and sighed deeply when she saw the box was gone. Entering her cell, she stopped and stared. Upon her bed sat her best-loved friend from childhood, a ragged bear with one missing eye. The acolyte picked him up and cuddled him, then carefully placed him against the pillows of her bed. Her spirit was lighter as she went off to say Night Prayer.

Demeter: A Spell to Increase
A Parent's Love

THE MATERIALS

- One geode. It may be whole and uncut, containing the mystery; or cut, revealing the treasure within. Your choice!

THE PURPOSE

The love we have for our children is indescribable. They are born of our bodies and thus are bonded to us beyond the life that we see. The act of beginning a child should be one of love, and as the child grows within we give over our bodies, thoughts, and feelings to the process, loving the *idea* of the child before it is even born. Men have a different experience of being a parent. Their seed went into the making of the child, but they miss that growing connection of their bodies to the child. However, many men do connect emotionally as their mates become a ripe and rounded vessel within which their child grows and draws nourishment. Sometimes when a couple joins for lovemaking a man may even feel a sort of physical connection with the babe.

The *idea* of the child is what makes a miscarriage or stillbirth so very difficult, for all of the tomorrows one expected to have with that particular child, accompanied with all the expectations and plans, are wiped away.

We tend to glorify mother-love as the almost magical "maternal instinct," when in reality it is actually a learning experience. The helplessness of the newborn babe and our physical response when our milk lets down continues the bond that many create with the child before it is born, but the rest is trial and error, and often plain hard work. And as we learn to nurture the child we learn, in a deeper way, how to nurture ourselves. This ability to nurture will extend beyond the child to others.

Mother-love and father-love are very real experiences. Without it the race would have vanished a long time ago. This spell is for the purpose of developing and increasing the love that is needed in order to parent a child.

THE AFFIRMATION

"The love I have for my child weathers all things, bears all things, and lives beyond the experience of life and death."

THE STONE

Geodes may come in any shape or size, but the most recognizable ones are round or egg-shaped. These shapes gave rise to the belief that geodes are symbols of fertility. Their cave or womblike interiors make them symbols of the Mother Goddess, and their shape reminds one of the rounded bellies of pregnant women. Their shape may also be likened to testicles, thus are linked to male fertility as well. From the outside geodes have a dull, rough exterior, not even hinting at the beauty that resides within. When cut or sliced open they may reveal brilliant beds of crystals—clear quartz and amethyst are the most common. When hollow, they may also contain milky water left over from their formation. If solid, they reveal beautiful patterns of minerals such as agate or jasper. Besides their use in promoting fertility, geodes may also be used to prevent miscarriage and for the successful birth of a child. A geode is an excellent stone to use to promote mother- or father-love.

THE GODDESS

Demeter is the Greek goddess of fertility and abundance. She was the Great Mother Goddess of the ancients. She and Her daughter Persephone were inextricably linked in both myths and rituals. Demeter lavished all of Her love on Her daughter, and the effects of that love were plenty and abundance of fields and groves. When Hades abducted Persephone and spirited Her away to the underworld, Demeter's grief and rage knew no end. She abandoned all in the search for Her daughter, even withdrawing the fruits of Her spirit. The land did not produce; all became as barren as Her grief rendered Her. It was not until the Gods became alarmed over the dying of the earth that they finally urged Zeus to intervene. He ordered that Persephone be released from the underworld and restored to Her mother. But since She had eaten a few seeds of the pomegranate offered by Hades, She was compelled to spend a part of the year with Him, away from Her mother. It is during this time that the land lays fallow, and the seed sleeps. However, with Her return Demeter's joy once again lends abundance to the earth, and all rejoice. This goddess, coupled with Her daughter, represents the cycle of life, death, and regeneration. Her single-minded love for Her daughter makes Her an ideal goddess to aid you in enhancing parental love.

THE MEDITATION (TO BE DONE IN CIRCLE)

You hold within your hands a round geode. It is rough and pregnant with possibilities. Shaking it, you hear liquid within; birth waters? The milk of life? You itch to slice it open to see what is hidden within. As you continue to hold it and gaze upon it, you feel yourself sinking into a trancelike state. Without becoming aware of it, you enter the rock you are holding. Like a cave with no opening, it is dark. You are not even sure *where* you are. Then a light is struck and it glances off of beds of brilliant crystals revealing all the colors of the rainbow. You are within the womb of the earth. Before you stands a goddess. She is holding a torch. She is dressed in robes of rich greens and gold. Her eyes are the brown of the lush, fertile earth, as is Her hair. She points at a bed of crystals at Her feet. Within them you see children. They are of all ages. They are of all the races of the world. They are whole and healthy, or infirm and disabled. But they are all loved, and they all live life to their fullest capabilities. Then the Goddess points to crystals that drip from the ceiling. Within them you see small lives never allowed to see the light of day, or those who had died during childhood of various causes. These souls are patiently awaiting rebirth, and play and romp together in the meadows of Summerland. You are then shown mothers and fathers from all places and all walks of life. They love their children as best they can, and though some fall far short in their loving, the Goddess blesses them, but cares for and protects their children as best She can. You understand that mother- and father-love is more complicated than you imagined, and you resolve to love those children in your care as purely as you can, and with the help of this goddess. You awake, still holding the geode in your hands. You take the lessons you have been shown deep within your heart, like the treasure within the geode, vowing to *be* Demeter to those in your care.

THE SPELL

Go to your ritual place. Set up your altar, cast your Circle, and request the presence of the Guardians. Invoke the goddess Demeter, and in the presence of All, bless your stone by air, fire, water, earth, and spirit. Sit quietly before your altar and, with stone in hand, engage in the meditation. Keep your affirmation—that the love you have for your child weathers all things, bears all things, and lives beyond the experience of life and death—clearly before you. At the conclusion of the meditation, when it feels right to you, stand before your altar and intone the spell, directing energy into your stone as you do so:

Mother is the cradle from which
we emerge to greet a world
both wide and delicious.

With primitive senses we explore—
touching, tasting, seeing, hearing, smelling—
mastering our environment;
becoming independent beings.

Mother is the cradle into which we fall
when at last we take our
final rest.

Mother-love surrounds us from
birth to beyond death.

The children of our heart
light up the dark
like the sun at midnight
or filaments of pure spirit.
Lady, may I ever respect
my child and embrace
her (him) with
love and security always.
So mote it be.

When ready, give thanks to All present for Their assistance. Open the Circle and Close the Temple.

Keep the geode either on your altar or in a place where you will see it often so you will be reminded of your role as Demeter to your child. It may be either cut open or left whole. If you choose to keep it whole, if ever there comes a time you wish to open it, pay attention to what is going on between you and your child. The curiosity to *know* what is inside may reflect some process going on in your relationship.

THE TIMING

This spell should be worked on a Monday just before the full moon. This symbolizes the fullness of love and care for your child, but recognizes that there is always room for more.

THE INCENSE

Myrrh. This incense presages death and loss, which Demeter certainly experienced, but also the joy of restoration and plenty.

THE CANDLES

White for purity of intention; pink for love; green for fertility and abundance.

THE PRACTICAL STEPS

- Before you can nurture your children, or others in your care for that matter, you must first nurture yourself. Do whatever it is that rejuvenates you: reading, walking the dog, gardening, writing in your journal, exercising, having lunch with a friend—whatever it is that is just for you. This is not being selfish; this is recharging your batteries so you may go out and *give* again.

- Meditate on what it means to be a mother or father. What do you think about it? What feelings do you have about it? What skills do you possess that make you a fit parent? What skills do you think you need? What are the joys and sorrows of parenthood? This meditation may help you appreciate what it means and takes to be a parent. Would you give it up if you could?

- Spend more "quality time" with each of your children. I know the phrase has been overused, but quality time is what you want to strive for. Do something the *child* wants to do: go to the park, the zoo, or even a favorite fast-food joint. After the activity perhaps the two of you could write or draw a story about your day.

Place it in your art gallery (the fridge door) and remember it together from time to time.

- Read to your child, and not just at bedtime: a rainy day before the fireplace with cocoa and miniature marshmallows is just perfect. This activity will encourage closeness, as well as teach your child to appreciate reading for fun. You can even do this with older children and teens. Let them choose the book, then take turns reading to each other. Enjoy the time together.

- Teach your child something you remember loving to do as a child. Get a telescope and stargaze together; plant a garden; begin a stamp or coin collection. Children are often fascinated by what their parents liked to do "when they were little." Try this and see if it opens up new vistas for your child. Seeing something "old" through a child's eyes is often a renewing experience for the adult as well.

- Eat your meals together, no matter how hectic schedules are. During mealtime ask about your child's day and really listen. Don't give advice or criticism, just use the time to get to know your child. You may also share aspects of your day depending on your child's age and attention span so he or she can get to know you. Never fight over "finishing your vegetables"; this only results in tears and upset.

- Always be positive with your child, even when you need to criticize or correct. Praise him or her for a job well done, or even for making a good effort. For esteem builders, create charts with stars and give monthly rewards, and send your child an occasional greeting card just to say "good job" or "I love you" so he or she can receive mail. Never call your child derogatory names or belittle him or her. And never hit. This teaches a child that physical violence is okay, and it produces bullies.

- Hug, kiss, and tell your child "I love you" often. A child learns what he or she lives. Teach your child to be affectionate both physically and verbally, but also teach him or her the difference between good and bad touching, and what to do if touched inappropriately.

THE PRIESTESS SPEAKS

The Priestess found the acolyte in a corner of the garden crying her eyes out. She gave the child her handkerchief and waited while she composed herself. Her voice thick with still unshed tears, and eyes downcast in embarrassment, the acolyte admitted to a bout of homesickness. The Priestess made a clucking sound and drew the girl to her ample bosom in a motherly hug, whereupon the girl began crying again. Later the other priestesses, on their way to Afternoon Prayer, found the Priestess gently rocking the girl and singing her a lullaby. The child, exhausted at last, had fallen asleep. Afternoon prayers could wait.

Yemoja: A Spell to Connect with Your Inner Child

THE MATERIALS

- A piece of coral. Traditionally, blue coral has been used to connect with one's inner child, but choose whatever color the child in you desires to use.

- A stand large enough for the coral to be displayed on.

THE PURPOSE

Isn't it a drag sometimes to always be the grown-up? We have all sorts of responsibilities clamoring for our time, all sorts of worries, all sorts of distasteful tasks that we must do in order to carry out the day-to-day process of living. Wouldn't it be nice to just say "No"? Well, this spell is for you. It is an opportunity to let go, just for awhile, of those onerous grown-up tasks and become a child again. Wanna go out and play? Do it! Wanna have ice cream for dinner? Go ahead! How about just whirling 'round and 'round until you get all dizzy and fall down laughing? Go for it! This spell will put you in touch with your inner child, who remembers how to play. He or she will touch you with magic so you may throw off the cares of the day and simply have good, childlike fun.

THE AFFIRMATION
"Ollie, Ollie Oxen free! I'm as happy as I can be!"

THE STONE
Coral are actually the remains of small sea creatures. After they die their tiny skeletons merge to become coral and, after years of this slow buildup, reefs are formed. Corals come in many shapes: branching, delicate rays of stars, mushroom, or appearing like small bushes, to name a few. They also come in many colors: red, blue, black, white, and shades of pink. Coral has been used traditionally to protect children from illness or as a general protection amulet. Pieces of coral were given to children to teethe on, or placed in rattles to make the sound. Since it is drawn from the sea it is also connected with the Mother Goddess. Because of its connection to children, as well as its many fun shapes and colors, coral is an appropriate stone to use to connect with your inner child.

THE GODDESS
Yemoja is a Nigerian Mother and Creator Goddess of the Yoruba tribe. She is connected with water, having created all of the waters in the area, as well as all bodies of saltwater. She gave birth to the sun and the moon, as well as to eleven other gods. When members of the Yoruba tribe were captured and taken away to various areas in the New World as slaves, their goddess went with them; She became known by many names and is even identified with the Virgin Mary. Yemoja is often depicted as a beautiful mermaid.

Mermaids have always fascinated me. As a child I even wanted to be one when I grew up! Mermaids depicted mystery, freedom, and an abundant capacity to play. Yemoja is a perfect goddess to call upon when you want to connect with the child-you.

THE MEDITATION (TO BE DONE IN CIRCLE)

You see yourself as a small naked person just floating, gently floating. You are surrounded by water; it is above you and below you. You are not afraid and you find you can breathe easily in this watery element. As you continue to float you can hear the heartbeat of the world reverberating through the waters. The resplendent song of whales accompanies it. You realize that this small naked person is actually the child-you that you lost touch with such a long time ago. You embrace him or her mentally and say "hi." You continue to gently drift with the current; the water is warm, like the waters of your mother's womb. Looking around you see coming toward you a creature out of legend. A beautiful mermaid is swimming lazily your way. Her skin is the color of roasted coffee beans, Her hair is black, and Her eyes are the color of midnight. Her gorgeous tail and fins are the color of green Chinese silk; Her headdress is of mother-of-pearl and decorated with colorful shells and bits of gold. She wears a necklace of black pearls and fish bones, and in one hand is a cowrie shell. She swims up to you; you reach out to touch Her, just to make sure She's real. She laughs, tiny bubbles escaping to the surface. Then She says, "Come, play with me." You follow Her, finding you can swim as easily as She can, and soon you are playing with dolphins and being dazzled by schools of tiny silver fish. You feel free and joyous, and spin and whirl through the water as gracefully as any sea creature. The goddess watches with a huge grin on Her lovely face. Finally She calls you to Her side. She holds out the shell that She has been carrying and gives it to you. It opens at your touch, and lying within is a lovely piece of coral, colorful and with an interesting shape. "This is for you to use whenever you need to leave tediousness behind and enter into the world of play," says the Goddess. You gratefully accept the gift and reluctantly depart this enchanted realm.

THE SPELL

Go to your ritual place. Set up your altar, cast your Circle, and request the presence of the Guardians. Invoke the goddess Yemoja, and in the presence of All, bless your stone by air, fire, water, earth, and spirit. Sit quietly before your altar and, with stone in hand, engage in the meditation. Keep your affirmation— "Ollie, Ollie, Oxen free, I'm as happy as I can be"—clearly before you. At the conclusion of the meditation, when it feels right to you, stand before your altar and intone the spell, directing energy into your stone as you do so:

> Yemoja:
> graceful goddess
> of the sea,
> exuberant and playful,
> Your laughter beckons
> to me like a
> siren's song—
> I drop my cares and burdens
> and attempt to sing along.
> Lovely Lady bedecked in
> coral and albescent pearls,
> I leap and frolic in
> thought and spirit,
> a child upon the golden
> sands of time.
> So mote it be.

When ready, give thanks to All present for Their assistance. Open the Circle and close the Temple.

Keep your coral on its stand and in a place where you will see it often. Pick it up and handle it, and while you do so recite the spell. Then go out and play!

THE TIMING

This spell should be worked on a Sunday just on or after the new moon.

THE INCENSE

Vanilla, coconut, or licorice. If you can find a scent that reminds you of your childhood—bubble gum or rain-washed pavement, for instance—use it. Some synthetic oils offer a whole range of scents from which to choose.

THE CANDLES

Get a selection of birthday candles. You may get the little plastic holders for them and stick them into a pot of earth, then the candles will be secure. Use a rainbow of colors, both solids and stripes, or get the ones that are in the shape of numbers, using the ones that represent your ideal childhood age.

THE PRACTICAL STEPS

- Meditate on your childhood in order to get in touch with your happy places. Not everyone had a carefree and loving childhood, so if yours was less than desirable let your imagination create a new one for you. What was it like? What did you enjoy and have fun doing? Think back and connect with that happy, playful child.

- Do something childlike. Get on the floor and play jacks or shoot marbles. Jump rope, not for exercise but for fun. Recite the rhymes you used as a child. Blow bubbles. Eat Pez candies. Make puppets from lunch bags. Watch Saturday morning cartoons in your jammies. Get out board games like Candy Land or Chutes and Ladders and draw in other childlike souls to play them with you. Laugh!

- Go to a park and swing on the swings, play on the jungle gym, and slide down the slide. If there's one of those small merry-go-rounds, get someone to push you as you lay on your back, watching the sky and clouds go 'round and 'round.

- Eat your favorite foods without worrying about calories. The smell and taste of these foods will take you back to your childhood.

- Go to the library, but bypass the adult section and head for the children's books. Check out some of your favorite childhood stories or pick out some new ones. Ask the librarian for help with some of the newer titles. Go home, make some cocoa with miniature marshmallows, and curl up and enjoy the books. Pay attention to the pictures and let your imagination roam.

THE PRIESTESS SPEAKS

It was the afternoon of a Holy Day and, except for the prescribed rituals, it was a day of rest and relaxation. The Priestess sat on the veranda with some of the other priestesses. All watched as the acolytes, freed from various duties today, frolicked and played on the wide lawns. With a sigh one of the priestesses commented on how much fun they seemed to be having. With a twinkle in her eyes the Priestess hiked up her robes, swatted one of her sisters on the arm, and cried "Tag. You're *it!*" Laughing, everyone got into the game. A good time was had by all.

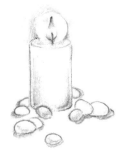

Nisaba: A Spell to Promote Dreaming

THE MATERIALS

- One rhodocrosite stone.

- A pouch made of soft but durable material. It may be pink to match your stone, or, if you can find it, purchase material with a motif of moon, stars, and night clouds.

THE PURPOSE

Sleep is the vessel of dreams, and dreams may foretell the future or shed light on the past. Our bodies require a certain amount of sleep in order to maintain physical, emotional, and psychological health. Dreams are part of that health. Without sleep and dreams people have been known to experience psychotic episodes.

Dreams may be full-fledged Technicolor movies or fragments, barely remembered upon waking. Common dream images have been defined in various ways, but they must still be considered to be idiosyncratic to the dreamer when attempting to interpret individual dreams. In times past dreams have been used in an attempt to achieve physical cures. Some cultures differentiate between "dream time" and "real time," and who's to say which is which?

Dreams are one way of connecting with our unconscious to get answers to our questions and deepen an understanding of our patterns and unacknowledged needs or desires. And they can be great entertainment!

THE AFFIRMATION

"My dreams bring healing and knowledge of self."

THE STONE

Rhodocrosite is a lovely stone in various shades of pink with bands of deep rose, white, and sometimes gray or black running through it. The name comes from the Greek *rhoddon* for rose, and *chroma* for color. This stone affects the emotions and may be used to clarify or balance them. It may affect the intuitive self, and has traditionally been used to enhance dream states. This is an excellent stone to use to promote dreaming.

THE GODDESS

Nisaba was the Sumerian goddess who gave Her people the gifts of reading and writing. She also imparted to them Her divine laws. She was an architect and appeared to the king in a dream in order to give him the specifications for a temple. She was an oracular goddess and interpreted dreams. Snakes, symbolic of transformation and regeneration, were associated with Her. She is an appropriate goddess to call upon for this spell.

THE MEDITATION (TO BE DONE IN CIRCLE)

You find yourself in a dream. It is a lovely dream. It feels safe and comfortable and happy. Take a moment now and allow your mind free rein to slip into a favorite daydream, one that makes you feel good. Build it up in your mind and simply enjoy it for a few moments (if you tape these meditations this would be a good place to insert some dreamy music you enjoy). After a few moments, let your daydream fade away. You are now floating among the stars; night clouds and the silver moon are your companions. You feel very peaceful. You notice the goddess Nisaba coming toward you, riding upon the back of a colorful serpent. Her robes are black and edged in silver. Her hair is black, caught up by a river of stars. Her eyes have endless depth. She soundlessly communicates to you, and you understand that She opens up the dream world to you. By entering this world at will you dip into your unconscious, and the Collective Unconscious of the universe. All knowledge, both past and present, is available to you. It may be used to better understand yourself, or to see how you fit within the "Big Picture." You may even have visions and prophesy, seeing future events from the all-seeing perspective of your dreams. These are great gifts, and you cherish them. Nisaba reaches out and plucks a rosy star from the deep night. It becomes a lovely rhodocrosite stone in Her hand. The goddess gives this to you and counsels you to place it beneath your pillow where it will aid you in your dreaming. You thank this goddess, and as this dream begins to tatter She sprinkles you with silver star dust and bids you to always have sweet dreams.

THE SPELL

Go to your ritual place. Set up your altar, cast your Circle, and request the presence of the Guardians. Invoke the goddess Nisaba, and in the presence of All, bless your stone by air, fire, water, earth, and spirit. Sit quietly before your altar and, with stone in hand, engage in the meditation. Keep your affirmation—that your dreams will bring healing and knowledge of your self—clearly before you. At the conclusion of the meditation, when it feels right to you, stand before your altar and intone the spell, directing energy into your stone as you do so:

> Nisaba,
> goddess of the dream,
> send to me

visions of power,
of knowledge.
I roam the dream world
at will and open
my inner eye,
unblinking in the truths
I find there.
Lady of the dream,
enfold me in Thy dark night
and let me dream again.
So mote it be.

When ready, give thanks to All present for Their assistance. Open the Circle and close the Temple.

Keep your rhodocrosite under your pillow when you want to dream and to remember your dreams. When not in use it should be kept in its pouch.

THE TIMING

This spell should be worked on a Monday when the moon is dark and the night is quiet.

THE INCENSE

Hyacinth, jasmine, lavender, or sweet pea. Other light floral scents that you enjoy may also be used.

THE CANDLES

Silver to connect to the moon, the unconscious, and visions, and dark blue for a peaceful, dreaming mind.

THE PRACTICAL STEPS

- Keep a dream journal and pen by your bed. Upon waking, even in the middle of the night, write down your dreams, or the images that you remember. Dreams tend to fade like morning mist, and often cannot be recalled even ten minutes after waking up.

- Now that you have captured your dreams you may take them individually or, when a pattern emerges, serially, and interpret them. First do some stream-of-consciousness writing. Let your ideas and images flow as you tell yourself a story about the dream. Then go ahead and consult a dream dictionary, as some of the definitions may pertain to your dream. Above all, have fun with this exercise.

- Share your dreams with a friend who is interested in interpreting dreams. First tell your friend what you think your dream means, then ask for feedback. Sometimes a fresh view might offer something valuable to your understanding. Then do the same for your friend.

- Draw or paint your dreams. Often the colors you choose to represent your dream will offer more information about the meaning of the dream. Don't worry about whether you can draw, just do it!

THE PRIESTESS SPEAKS

Goddess House was quiet beneath an ebony sky scattered with a dusting of stars. Everyone was asleep. The Priestess glided quietly through the house. Her sight tested the flavor of the sleeper's dreams, and where she found anxiety or even a nightmare she sent soothing thoughts. The Priestess, Weaver of Dreams, was satisfied that her charges were well.

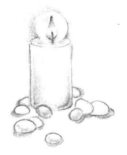

Hecate: A Spell to Celebrate Menopause

THE MATERIALS

- Jet. This may be a single piece, or several beads or chips made into a necklace.

- A black pouch made of soft but durable material in which to keep the piece(s) when not in use.

THE PURPOSE

Images of the Crone bring up an old, wizened woman wrapped in a black cape, hair grizzled and gray, eyes like raisins sunk into doughy flesh. She is hunched over due to the hump she carries on her back, and she needs a stick to both help her keep her balance and to beat off yapping dogs and small children. She cackles when she laughs and smells of the cabbages she cooks. She is thoroughly unpleasant and a little mad.

These images of the Crone have found their way into fairy tales and the Collective Unconscious of the planet. This negative Crone has nothing to redeem her in our thoughts and engenders only disgust and fear. But there is another Crone behind this unlovely caricature. She is a Lady of wisdom, mystery, and magic. She meets you at the crossroads and unfolds your destiny before you. She is the destroyer, and clears the way for regeneration and new growth. She holds life and death in the balance, and leads the soul into the underworld and what lies beyond. She guides the self to inner seeing and understanding; integration is Her prize.

Menopause is a time when, like adolescence, we find our body is off doing its own thing, dragging our thoughts and emotions unwillingly in its wake. We are moving from the rich fertile woman with childbearing possibilities to the rich fertile woman of ancient wisdom. The "children" of this time are of the mind and of the heart. Through the process of menopause when our blood courses run dry, we enter into the Dark Mother's cycle and are hidden beneath a black moon. This can be both a frightening and a freeing time; frightening because we are in the process of becoming someone entirely different from what we were before, with different roles and expectations; freeing in that we may become whatever we want to become, with no restrictions or limitations. Menopause should be viewed as a right of passage, and post-menopausal women honored as Crones of wisdom, mystery, and magic.

THE AFFIRMATION

"I am an empty vessel filled by the Goddess."

THE STONE

Jet is actually fossilized wood created millions of years ago. It is usually a dark brown or black, and has a waxy finish to it. It is a surprisingly light stone in weight, so it should be purchased from a reputable source or you might end up with a product made from plastic. Traditionally it has been used for protection and to absorb negative energies. It may be used to guard against nightmares, and to enhance psychic and divinatory processes. Jet, coupled with amber, has been worn when calling upon the Goddess. It has a connection to the chthonic world and thus to the Crone, opening up the gates to the unconscious and laying before the seeker the road to the inner self. It is an excellent stone to use to embrace the deeper, darker self revealed by the menopausal process.

THE GODDESS

Hecate was originally a Thracian goddess but was incorporated into the classical Greek pantheon, though She seemed always to take on a life of Her own and reveal depths of Herself to those who came to know Her. She is a Triple Goddess: of the heavens, the earth, and the underworld, and also of the triple phases of the moon—new, full, and dark (or Maiden, Mother, and Crone). As the moon She was Hecate Selene, Artemis, the hunter on earth, and Persephone, queen of the underworld. She can be found at the crossroads where three roads meet, and there unfolds your destiny if you are brave enough to look for it. She is a goddess of mystery, magic, and wisdom, and most often presents Herself as the Crone, the post-menopausal woman of power. She is an excellent goddess to invoke for this spell.

THE MEDITATION (TO BE DONE IN CIRCLE)

You find yourself before a large black cauldron. It is filled with clear spring water. It is night, and the sky is a black curtain spotted with winking silver stars. There is no moon. The air is chilly and the scent of autumn is in the air. A great raven with outstretched wings flies toward you and as you watch, it coalesces into mist and then into a woman of indeterminate age. Her hair is a river of silver and Her eyes are dark and knowing pools that reflect nothing and draw in everything. Her voluminous robes stir though there is no breeze. She says nothing, simply points into the cauldron. You allow your gaze to settle on the water, which turns an inky black without reflection. As you watch you see yourself, a woman of mature years, a woman who now feels the fires moving rampant in her body as the rivers of life recede. You are frightened at these changes, yet also curious to see what will be left, what will be fashioned of this empty vessel. Pictures unfold of your wise self, your magical self, your divine self. You know you will be different, but also stronger and more fully and truly yourself, as now you may allow the Divine to fill you up. The flow is not of blood but of the sacred, and you are at peace. Hecate removes a stone from Her hair, a piece of jet. This stone will remind you of your ongoing transformation, and of Her presence in your life from now on.

THE SPELL

Go to your ritual place. Set up your altar, cast your Circle, and request the presence of the Guardians. Invoke the goddess Hecate, and in the presence of All, bless your stones by air, fire, water, earth, and spirit. Sit quietly before your altar and, with stones in hand, engage in the meditation. Keep your affirmation—that you are an empty vessel filled by the Goddess—clearly before you. At the conclusion of the meditation, when it feels right to you, stand before your altar and intone the spell, directing energy into your stones as you do so:

> Hecate, Lady of the Night,
> great raven with
> outstretched wings,
> mistress of mystery
> and magic,
> You lead me to the crossroads
> of my desire and
> envelop me in Your darkness.
> Silently You lead the way;
> darkness and solitude are
> my only companions.
> Into the depths we go,
> until my senses fail
> and I stand,
> revealed and trembling;
> my fragmented self
> becomes whole,
> and I take my place as Your
> blessed companion.
> So mote it be.

When ready, give thanks to All present for Their assistance. Open the Circle and close the Temple.

As you go through the menopausal process with all of its physical, emotional, and mental challenges and changes, carry or wear your jet. Feel your connection with the Crone, and realize that you are not losing anything of value; on the contrary, you are gaining an identity of self unfettered by useless and worn out beliefs and activities. Your path is as clear as Hecate's dark reflective eyes.

THE TIMING

This spell is best worked on a Monday or a Saturday, if possible, just before the new moon, when the moon hides Her face and opens a door to the underworld.

THE INCENSE

Cypress, myrrh, or sandalwood.

THE CANDLES

Black for the Dark Mother and the darkened moon; red for the blood we shed. After the red candle has burned down completely (and safely), its stub should be buried in rich earth where it will not be disturbed.

THE PRACTICAL STEPS

- Go to the library and check out a book such as *Our Bodies, Ourselves for the New Century: A Book by and for Women*. Educate yourself about what the process of menopause is all about— not just the physical aspects, but the cultural and emotional aspects as well.

- Find a health care professional with whom you feel comfortable and who is willing to really talk with you about the changes your body will go through as well as all of the options available to you for management, even the adjunctive (alternative) treatments. There are ways to make the passage less uncomfortable.

- Join a support group. Being with other women who are going through the same thing can be very uplifting. If you can't find one, start one!

- Create a ritual to acknowledge your change of status from childbearing woman to wise woman. Your children will now be the wisdom you have to share with others in your world.

- You may find that your dreams and meditations may be strange or very different now. Pay attention to these, for they will reveal truths you need right at this time.

- This is a time when you may feel very free sexually. Write, draw, paint, or sculpt what that freedom is like. Embrace your sexuality and enjoy being a sensual woman. Always practice safe sex, but allow yourself to fly.

- As women grow older, and especially when menopause looms, we often fear a loss of our youthful looks. Do a journal exercise. Write "I am beautiful when . . ." Come up with at least ten items for your list. Our beauty resides in more than just our looks.

THE PRIESTESS SPEAKS

The night is dark with only the stars for celestial company. The Priestess stands within the Circle and invites a priestess to enter. The acolyte precedes her, carrying an empty cauldron, which she places before the Priestess' feet. This sister is making the transition from Mother to Crone within the community, as her blood courses have stopped flowing. The ceremony is simple; the Priestess lifts the empty cauldron to the heavens, and when She presents it to her sister, it is full of light. The new Crone deeply inhales this light and is filled; the gates of wisdom open, and she now takes her place with the Counsels of the Wise.

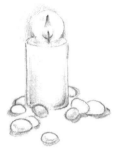

Eriskegal: A Spell for Confronting Death

THE MATERIALS

- Obsidian, a natural stone; choose a size appropriate for scrying.

- A black pouch made of soft but durable material in which to keep the stone when not in use.

THE PURPOSE

Death. What does that word evoke for you? Does it cause a shiver to run up and down your spine? Do you feel a thrill of fear? Of protest or revulsion? Is there a sense of curiosity, of wonder? Does it cause you to remember the loss of someone close to you, or of a beloved pet? For many people death is something we don't think about unless it touches us personally. Death is something we deny consciously, but which lurks in our unconscious; it is the knowledge that someday we, too, will die.

How does one cope with that knowledge? Some find that their religious or spiritual beliefs hold out the hope that there is something beyond this life; that when our lives wind down and end and our souls flee the darkened flesh, the "I" of our existence continues in some other place, in some other form. Some people simply refuse to acknowledge the hold that death, from the very moment of our birth, has over us. They are those who will not go gently into that dark night, but will fight it every step of the way. And then there are those who accept death's reality but determine to live fully until it is their time to go, thus wholly appreciating the gift of their lives.

Whatever your beliefs, this spell is for the purpose of facing the knowledge of death so that we may continue in life with a greater appreciation for every breath we take.

THE AFFIRMATION

"Death is but the gateway to life."

THE STONE

Obsidian is actually volcanic glass, formed by molten lava that cooled before crystals could form. Most obsidian is black, but some may be found in various shades of gray with some rare deposits of red, blue, and green. Obsidian may be used for grounding and absorbing negative energies. It is a revelatory stone, bringing to light that which is hidden and making way for transformation. It enhances meditation and can take the seeker into that central silence needed for inner seeing. Its shiny black surface has been used for scrying. It will open doors to the unconscious, sometimes revealing things that we may not feel ready to face. This stone has depths within depths, and is an excellent one to use when confronting one's feelings about death.

THE GODDESS

Eriskegal was the Sumerian goddess of the underworld. She originally ruled this realm alone until the god Nergal was introduced by patriarchal forces. Nevertheless, it was Eriskegal who shared Her throne with Him. Eriskegal welcomed the dead into Herself, releasing them from the toils of life and giving them rest. As goddess even over life She caused Her sister Inanna, queen of heaven, to die, but then restored Her to the living. This goddess is appropriate to call upon when dealing with issues of death, that journey that awaits us all.

THE MEDITATION (TO BE DONE IN CIRCLE)

You find yourself in a watery womb. You feel safe, warm, loved. You cannot see. You cannot hear. You cannot speak. You simply feel the liquid warmth surrounding you, supporting you. Then, faintly, you hear a heartbeat. Soft and rhythmic, it enters you and your heart begins to beat to this other's rhythm. As you listen to the beat, ensconced in this pleasant womb, you are gently ferried to a dark shore. Once there a naked, black-haired woman meets you. She lifts you from the water and leads you to dry shore. You find you cannot gaze into Her eyes too long, for there are depths there in which you will become lost. Eriskegal, goddess of death, of the underworld, makes you welcome to Her realm. It is not at all what you expected; it is more wonderful than any of your fantasies or hidden dreams. You wonder why you feared to take death's path. The mysteries of your heart unfold before you and you find a sense of peace that escaped you in life. All of the lessons of your life are suddenly so clear, and the seasons of regret, of pain you may have felt or have caused others, of disappointments, flash away in Eriskegal's dark eyes. You are whole and complete at last. You realize that death is a friend and guide, and you eagerly open to Her secrets. Fear is gone. You vaguely realize that this is a dream, and in order to remember it Eriskegal gives you a piece of obsidian that adorned Her hair. Its glassy black surface will return you to Her realm whenever you scry into it. You return to the land of the living; by knowing death you may live your life more fully and with greater zest.

THE SPELL

Go to your ritual place. Set up your altar, cast your Circle, and request the presence of the Guardians. Invoke the goddess

Eriskegal, and in the presence of All, bless your stone by air, fire, water, earth, and spirit. Sit quietly before your altar and, with stone in hand, engage in the meditation. Keep your affirmation—that death is but the gateway to life—clearly before you. At the conclusion of the meditation, when it feels right to you, stand before your altar and intone the spell, directing energy into your stone as you do so:

> The velvet darkness of death
> embraces the soul,
> released from life's fleshy hold.
> Journeys end and begin
> with the exhale of a breath.
> The unbound compassion of the Goddess
> flows with soothing grace
> around the soul and guides
> her to a place of
> respite and release.
> Eriskegal tenderly
> contains the essence;
> I will have no fear when
> I step through the gateway of death.
> So mote it be.

When ready, give thanks to All present for Their assistance. Open the Circle and close the Temple.

Use your obsidian as a scrying stone whenever questions of death, transformation, and release present themselves to you. Let the stone reveal the answers you seek. Give thanks to the Goddess for Her intervention and guidance. If facing death due to illness this spell will offer you a way to release your anxieties about dying. The stone will offer visions of the life to come. If facing the loss of someone you love, it will calm your fears about being left behind, while allowing you to let go of that person's mortality while appreciating his or her immortal self.

THE TIMING

This spell should be worked on a Saturday during a waning moon.

THE INCENSE

Frankincense, myrrh, or patchouli.

THE CANDLES

Black: all absorbing; the symbol of the pervasive nothingness of death that leads to life.

THE PRACTICAL STEPS

- For many reasons, it is important to understand your attitudes toward death. Knowing your beliefs about death and dying is important for living your life. Our feelings about death can reveal how we approach all the facets of our living. Engage in journal writing to explore this overlooked area of your life. Pay attention to dreams. Begin to develop your own philosophy of death, and what it means to you.

- Go to the library and check out some books about death and dying. Start with children's books such as *The Next Place* by War- ren Hanson or *The Fall of Freddie the Leaf: A Story of Life for All Ages* by Leo Buscaglia. These books are full of wisdom and will connect with your unconscious thoughts about death, opening up a path of fruitful contemplation.

- Write a eulogy for your own funeral. How do you want to be remembered? Does your eulogy match with who you are and what you are doing today? Do you need to make any changes in order to become the person you want others to remember? This experience will give you food for thought and may bring up some uncomfortable feelings. Try to go with them and let them unfold.

- Engage in some volunteer work having to do with death and dying. Become a hospice volunteer and work with people who are completing the process of their living. This can be a scary thing to do, but people who are on this journey have much to teach. Simply be present, listen, and offer compassionate care and attention. The riches you will receive cannot be counted.

THE PRIESTESS SPEAKS

The community stood in Circle beneath a waning moon. One of their members entered death's realm today. The Priestess, dressed all in black, raises her hands to the sky and begins the prayer. Her face shines with an inner light, and joy spills from her eyes. She knows that death is but a gateway, and holds no fear. The acolyte, crying over the lost one, looks with wonder at the Priestess and feels a fiery bolt of hope, an understanding of depths beyond depths. She, too, may now release her sister with joy.

Arianrhod: A Spell for Preparation for Rebirth

THE MATERIALS

- Rhodonite stones. These should be a collection of separate polished stones. Choose a number that speaks to you, but make sure there are seven or more.

- A pouch made of soft but durable material, either black or a color that matches your stones.

THE PURPOSE

In Wiccan and other Pagan belief systems we are not simply single bright candles against the darkness, but rather we shine multiple times. The Wheel of the Year may be seen as a *type* or metaphor for the countless cycles of birth, death, and rebirth that we experience. We move through the lessons of our lives, adding wisdom, understanding, compassion, wonder, and love to each one until we are absorbed into the All-Mother/All-Father, embraced by the Light of Sacred Spirit. As we move around the Wheel we become more and more aware of our own connection with Divinity, of the very real fact that Goddess and God shine from our eyes and embrace the world with our hands.

Death comes before rebirth, and thus is midwife to each new life. What has gone before often sets the pattern for what will come, and each new experience is just that. Each pristine life becomes a promise of awareness and delight, if we are but open to it. Life is a garden that we tend, well or poorly or somewhere in between. We should pay attention to that which we plant, and determine to produce the best fruits we are capable of.

This spell is for the purpose of opening to the possibilities. We may have fantasies of "life as it should be"; this spell is to get us thinking about what we want, not only for the future *now*, but for that far distant shore that is as yet indistinct—the realm of potential.

THE AFFIRMATION

"I embrace my future self by tending well the garden I plant now."

THE STONE

Rhodonite is a lovely opaque stone that is deep rose in color with black, brown, or gray markings throughout. The stones that are rose and gray or rose and black are especially striking. This stone has been used to decrease anxiety, to ground and balance, and to clear the psychic centers. Just holding it helps me to relax and *breathe*. It gives me a sense of well-being. This stone called out to be used for this spell, and since it works on the psychic centers and has the other attributes mentioned, it is appropriate to use.

THE GODDESS

Arianrhod is a Welsh goddess who resides in Caer Arianrhod or Castle Arianrhod. Her name means "Silver Wheel," and She is connected to the circumpolar stars that never set. There, souls are drawn after physical death to await rebirth. As with many goddess types, this goddess has a triple aspect: Arianrhod the Initiator; Blodeuwedd the Nurturer; and Cerridwen, the White Sow who destroys our flesh even as the soul flees it, freeing us for new beginnings. This goddess takes us into Her realm and prepares us for rebirth, acting as a midwife as we enter into our next life. She is an excellent goddess to call upon in order to meditate upon the possibilities of our future lives.

THE MEDITATION (TO BE DONE IN CIRCLE)

You are floating in a dark sky surrounded by a ring of fire. The fire separates itself into distinct balls of brilliant light, resolving into individual stars. They pulsate to the rhythm of the universe, and are of every imaginable color. You are dazzled by their beauty and warmed by their passionate fire. As you watch them dance around you, you notice a lovely woman coming toward you. Her hair is like black night and Her eyes are a brilliant blue, like twin flames. Upon Her hair is a diadem of stars no less bright than those that surround you. You feel joy just looking at Her, and She smiles at you and takes your hand. You are so full of light that you join Her in the dance, and as you do She imparts to you flashing visions of possibilities of future lives to live. (At this point take some time to allow the visions to come.) The Silver Wheel burns bright with each choice, and you know that you *do* have a choice. The lessons are yours to seek out, and Arianrhod will open the gates of life once again in order for you to plunge joyfully into the passionate life you choose. However, She cautions you to tend your current garden well, or these choices may fade like morning mist, with others growing in their stead. But all are necessary and all are useful; it is simply a matter of what you do with them that matters. After reviewing the possibilities Arianrhod gives you several lovely rose and black stones in order to remind you to live a balanced, compassionate, and joyful life. You may leave all anxieties aside as you return to your current house of flesh, knowing that you will live more thoughtfully and pay attention to the lessons that come your way.

THE SPELL

Go to your ritual place. Set up your altar, cast your Circle, and request the presence of the Guardians. Invoke the goddess Arianrhod, and in the presence of All, bless your stones by air, fire, water, earth, and spirit. Sit quietly before your altar and, with stones in hand, engage in the meditation. Keep your affirmation—to embrace your future self by tending your current garden well—clearly before you. At the conclusion of the meditation, when it feels right to you, stand before your altar and intone the spell, directing energy into your stones as you do so:

> The soul retreats and
> flees the flesh;
> humanity's cloak no longer needed.
> The stars call to the eager
> soul and act as beacons to guide
> her home.
>
> Arianrhod, sweet goddess
> of respite,
> You welcome the weary traveler
> within Your castle bright.
> The soul asks but a moment
> before journeying on again.
>
> As the stars turn so do the seasons,
> and they capture once again the
> soul's imagination.
> Flexing her intentions,
> she plunges like light
> into the world again.
>
> Arianrhod watches over all.
> Bright goddess guide me well.
> So mote it be.

When ready, give thanks to All present for Their assistance. Open the Circle and close the Temple.

Your stones may be used as indicators of past lives or current signposts. Meditate upon a question or issue you are struggling with and cast your stones upon your altar. While still in a meditative state divine the shapes that the scatter of stones form. Let images come to your mind, and allow your subconscious to unfold any meanings therein.

When not in use your stones should be kept in their pouch.

THE TIMING

This spell is best worked on a Monday just after a new moon.

THE INCENSE

Jasmine, lemon balm, or sandalwood.

THE CANDLES

White for guidance within the dark, and silver to connect with Caer Arianrhod, the castle made of brilliant stars.

THE PRACTICAL STEPS

- For more information about reincarnation go to your local library. Many cultures have believed in some form of reincarnation for centuries, and even early Christianity had room for the idea. It is certainly not new, and if the idea resonates with you it may be because you recognize the truth of this for you.

- Pay attention to déjà vu experiences. Former lessons not fully learned, or those important people with whom we need to connect again are often introduced to us through this mechanism. These are "must attend to" people and experiences, and will tend to add formation to future lives.

- Get involved with a meditation group or, better yet, a drumming circle or a group that participates in some form of ecstatic dancing. The rhythm of the drums often calls up interesting meditations of their own, and ecstatic dancing can open a flood of feelings and memories. You may experience a past life or receive insight into how to better live this one. Everything is part of the Wheel of past, present, and future. The drums or dancing may speak to you.

- Do some journal writing or create art depicting your life to date. Include those things you are proud of, and those things you may have some regret or shame over. Be honest about those times you could have done better, but be especially honest about your accomplishments. Include your compassionate activities on behalf of others and those times you took special care of yourself during difficult times.

- Now that you have a bit of your life to work from, look objectively through your journal or at your artwork. How can you take the lessons of your life, incorporate them into your current situation, and live more fully, more compassionately, and more genuinely? Make a list of how you can become more Divine, then work toward that goal.

- As always, pay attention to your dreams. They will give you clues as to changes you need to make, or issues that you need to pay attention to. They may also reveal bits and pieces of past lives that you need to be aware of for a current situation, or may offer a signpost for the future.

THE PRIESTESS SPEAKS

The Priestess stands alone among the stones. The night is black. Suddenly stars descend from the heavens and surround her. She reaches out and weaves them into the likeness of a chariot drawn by two adamantine steeds. Then she patiently waits. A moment passes, then two. A shining form takes place out of the darkness and drifts toward her. It flames bright with fierce vitality. Gently the Priestess hands this lucid soul into the waiting chariot and sends it skyward. A soul has passed this night from life to death. The Priestess, midwife of all, has sent her home to rest and take her joy until the Wheel rolls around and calls her back into the world.

Part Three

Invoking the Goddess/Invoking the God

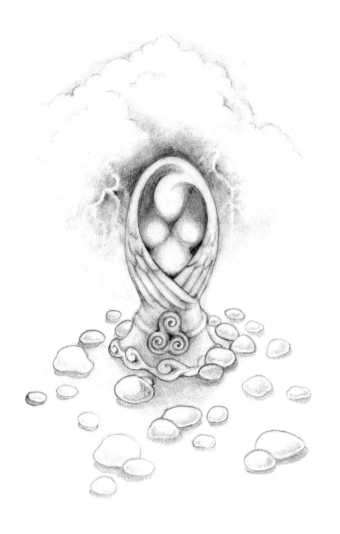

Embracing the Goddess

THE MATERIALS

- Amber. This may be in the form of a ring or necklace. A necklace of beads is preferable.

THE PURPOSE

This Goddess has no name or face. She is simply the Goddess. She is not bound by our need to describe Her or to capture Her with a name. She may be seen in the actions of the winds. She is the heart of the flame. The waters are Her lifeblood and the earth is Her bones. She is as elusive as star shine or as present as your beloved one. The ever-changing moon gives you a sense of Her; the fiery sun symbolizes the passion of Her love for you. She is approachable and nurturing to Her children, but She is also remote and mysterious. She gives life but is also the death-bringer, offering transformative initiation as Her gift.

The Goddess has been worshiped for millennia. As early as seven thousand years before the birth of Christ She was worshiped in Her threefold forms of Maiden, Mother, and Crone. She has been honored in every culture; only Her sacred names have changed, blossoming into a thousand-petaled flower. She is worshiped today, again in many cultures, many forms, and under myriad names. But all are one and are absorbed into the Nameless One, who is timeless.

We seek the Goddess because She, along with Her consort, the God, offers the embodiment of fullness. We seek the Goddess as a reflection of our feminine self. As nature strives for balance, so too in the spiritual realm do we find the balance of the feminine and masculine. Women may connect with the Goddess through their fertile, fecund bodies, their creative minds and spirits, and the paths of the unconscious. Men may reach Her by opening to their *anima*, the feminine aspect and guide of their inner self who leads them to their center and thus to Deity. Both men and women may experience the Goddess and the God through the avenue of love, cherishing each other and surrendering to love's embrace.

The Goddess, once aroused, will not meekly return to sleep. She will reveal possibilities undreamed of and will guide you into the deeper chambers of your soul. Embrace the Goddess and know peace.

THE AFFIRMATION

"Embracing the Goddess I am filled with Her light."

THE STONE

Amber is a magical substance. It is actually the product of coniferous tree resins that have been transformed by time into an organic stone. Its color may range from clear yellow to a rich golden-brown to a honey-red. It often has air bubbles trapped within it, bits of fern or other material from the tree that formed it, or even tiny insects who became caught within the sticky substance and were preserved there. Amber is warm to the touch and seems to have a life of its own. By rubbing it against cloth it can hold a small electric charge. Amber has a strong connection to the Goddess and is used by witches during meditation in order to help them become more in tune with Her. Amber is also used in magic to strengthen any spell. It attracts love, money, or other desirable things into one's life. It may be used in protection spells and is supposedly useful in a variety of healing spells. This is an appropriate stone to use in your quest of the Goddess.

THE GODDESS

Any Goddess-form may be used for this meditation and spell. You may call upon one with whom you are well acquainted, or extend your knowledge of Her by exploring how other people may have called upon and related to Her. Or you may simply call upon the Goddess, and allow Her to reveal Herself to you in the guise of Her choosing.

THE MEDITATION (TO BE DONE IN CIRCLE)

You dream. And within your dream you see your self, that part of you who is connected with Divinity; who *is* Divinity. In your dream you become this other self, or she becomes you. You move with liquid grace, traversing lands both well known and strange. Grass tickles bare feet; animals talk to you in half-remembered languages; the mountains' crashing laughter catapults you into shining, singing rivers. You lift a graceful arm and rise upon the air, dancing with dragonflies and sunbeams. The moon comes out in the middle of the day, and from her shining surface a chariot follows a path of light to earth. Driving it is Goddess, dressed all in white. She is ever-changing; the eye cannot behold Her for any longer than a moment, for She transforms within a blink. She invites you to join Her on the chariot's platform. Once there, She directs Her milky steeds to rise, and takes you on a whirlwind of a ride, revealing to you spiritual truths whose knowingness you now need. She traps each and every one within amber beads and strings them on a silver chain for you to wear. "Remember," She breathes, as She tumbles you from the chariot and back into your bed. You awaken with the Goddess within you, Her truths clutched in your hand.

THE SPELL

Go to your ritual place. Set up your altar, cast your Circle, and request the presence of the Guardians. Invoke the Goddess by whatever name (or no name) seems good to you, and in the presence of All, bless your stone(s) by air, fire, water, earth, and spirit. Sit quietly before your altar and, with stone(s) in hand, engage in the meditation. Keep your affirmation—to embrace the Goddess and thus be filled with Her light—clearly before you. At the conclusion of the meditation, when it feels right to you, stand before your altar and intone the spell, directing energy into your stone(s) as you do so:

> Great Goddess of
> the Night,
> within the obscuring darkness
> Your all-pervasive light
> stands first to guard us, then
> to be our guide,
> as we seek to know Thee,
> and within Thy sheltering heart abide.
>
> Lovely Lady of
> the day,
> who doth intermingle
> sorrow in Your play,
> remind us that within
> life shelters death;
> and that beyond the veil
> we grasp again ecstatic breath.
>
> Living goddess of
> moon and stream,

of eagle's flight and
growing grain,
bless this, Thy Priest(ess)
with Thine Art,
and hold me gently in
Thine heart.
So mote it be.

When ready, give thanks to All present for Their assistance. Open the Circle and close the Temple.

You should wear you amber beads or ring whenever possible in order to maintain the connection with the Goddess. When this is not possible, place them upon your altar. You may sleep with them under your pillow for pleasant, or revealing, dreams.

THE TIMING

This spell should be worked on a Monday at the time of the full moon. For the hidden aspects of the Goddess, or for the Crone, it may be worked during the dark of the moon. For the experience of Her Maiden-self, new moon is best.

THE INCENSE

Gardenia, honeysuckle, jasmine, lavender, lilac, rose, sweet pea, or any sweet-smelling scent you enjoy. You may also wear your favorite perfume as you perform this rite.

THE CANDLES

The colors of the Goddess are white for the Maiden, red for the Mother, and black for the Crone. For the Goddess in general, use silver candles for Her connection with the moon.

THE PRACTICAL STEPS

- Go to a place of nature where you are safe and comfortable. Sit and be still. Notice the plants around you, their type, size, shape, and colors. Be aware of the scent of the earth. Notice the creatures nearby—birds, insects, lizards, and any others. Watch them watching you! Experience the feel of the breeze against your skin, or how it plays with your hair and clothes. Taste the sky. Now take a deep breath and know that Goddess is nearby; She is within you.

- Meditate upon the Goddess. You may begin with a well-loved image, but as you sink into deeper realms of thought and experience, the image may shift and change. This is the Goddess showing Her true face to you. This, too, may change with successive meditations; Goddess is as changeable as the moon but as ever-present.

- Pray to the Goddess. Seek Her out within your heart. You are created in Her image. What does that make you?

- Create your very own goddess image for your altar through painting, sculpture, or another artistic medium. Make this a personal image, adding symbols or such things as stones, shells, dried flowers, or other found items to the piece. This is more than a creative exercise; through the art of creating, a deeper understanding of Goddess may be had.

- Give some thought to how the women in your life—daughter, mother, sister, lover—fulfill the various roles of the Goddess for you. Can you see the Divine within these special people? Do you feel differently about them knowing the Goddess may look at you from their eyes? By seeing the Divinity within, you may have a different appreciation for these women.

- Record your dreams, for often it is through dreaming that the Goddess speaks to us.

THE PRIESTESS SPEAKS

The acolyte, deep in prayer, does not hear the Priestess enter the Temple. Something prompts the girl to open vision-clouded eyes and She sees the Priestess at the altar, a rapture of light and glory. With a cry of "Lady" the acolyte flings herself at the Priestess' feet. The Priestess raises the girl with a smile and winking eyes, and places her finger before the girl's lips in the age-old symbol for "silence." She then turns and walks away, leaving the acolyte staring with mouth agape.

Embracing the God

THE MATERIALS

- Any God stone, such as sunstone, moss agate or fire agate, red jasper, garnet, ruby, topaz, citrine, tiger-eye, or smoky quartz. You may also use beads made of bone or antler, as long as these items were obtained from animals that died a natural and humane death.

THE PURPOSE

Life and death. Joy and sorrow. Day and night. Male and female. Everywhere we look this world is made up of pairs of opposites. Without one of these pairs the others would lose meaning and definition. We hold within us life, but also the seeds of death. We know joy and experience sorrow. We acknowledge the passage of time and of the seasons. Within all of us there resides masculine and feminine energies and attributes that reflect the greater forces of the universe, of Goddess and God.

As played out in myth and daily experience the God-form may be apprehended in many ways. He is the babe born anew at Winter Solstice, bringing light and hope into the world. He is the Young Lord in the fullness of His strength pursuing the elusive deer within the forest, courting the Spring Maiden as She dances flirtatiously before Him. He is the Mystic Lover, the Bridegroom, and the successful Hunter of the Moon who beds His Bride with lust and laughter. He is the Sacrifice, dying as the grain is cut so that we may live. He is the One whose passing we mourn with sorrow and lamentation and unbearable grief. In some cultures or traditions He has been portrayed as the loving Father who embraces all of His children, or the Good Shepherd who carries us when we can go no further.

All of these images give us a sense of the God. All of them are worthy of meditation and contemplation and allow us to enter into a deeper relationship with Him. Choose those facets that resonate with you and embrace Him, knowing that He is ever ready to partner us in the eternal dance of life.

THE AFFIRMATION

"I embrace the God; the God embraces me. I am whole."

THE STONE

For this meditation and spell you may choose any stone that speaks to you. It may be one you were particularly drawn to in an earlier section of this book, even one that was utilized for a specific "feminine" purpose, as within the heart of each stone is a bit of both masculine and feminine energies. Don't worry about whether or not you are familiar with or know any specifics about the stone you use. Let it choose you, and listen to what it says. It will be your personal link to the God in this spell, and a reminder of His presence in your life.

THE GOD

You may work with any God-form you like for this meditation and spell. You may call upon a particular image or attribute. You may call upon one you are familiar with, or you may expand your knowledge of the God-forms of other cultures and traditions by learning about a God-form new to you. You might just allow the meditation to take you to the throne of God, and let Him show Himself to you as He wishes.

THE MEDITATION (TO BE DONE IN CIRCLE)

You are in deep, virgin forest. No one has penetrated here before. The trees assault your eyes with the lushness of their greens. Their bark and the rich earth are shades of brown that you have never before seen. Wildflowers of every kind and color grow among the trees, offering a feast of beauty for your eyes. You are dressed and draped in these flowers, and your hair is crowned with sunlight. A hidden stream can be heard bubbling nearby, and birds of every sort sing competing songs among the branches. You revel in this wilderness, and feel comfortably at ease. Suddenly you hear the dulcet tones of a hunting horn. The birds fall instantly silent. Through the underbrush you hear the scrambling sound of an animal. You remain still, hardly breathing, as it is coming toward you. Without any further warning a white hart bursts from out of the trees. She is winded, breathing hard. You cannot help but notice that her eyes are like molten silver. She startles at the sight of you, then leaps beyond you and disappears into the deeper protection of the trees. You let go your breath, but upon the heels of the magnificent beast comes a Hunter. He is clad in leather and skins. His hair, dark and unruly, curls about His face. He stops His progress at the sight of you; the gaze He turns on you is sharp and intent. Then He smiles. His lips are full and sensual, and as you gaze at Him you are captured by His eyes, green flecked with gold. He lays aside His horn, His bow, and his quiver full of arrows, and comes to you, slowly, gently, as if He is afraid that you will run away, like the hart. As he reaches you He drops to one knee and extends His hand to you, palm up. "Lady," He says. You tentatively reach out to Him. Then you take His hand and raise Him to His feet. With one fluid motion He embraces you and carries you off into the forest.

THE SPELL

Go to your ritual place. Set up your altar, cast your Circle, and request the presence of the Guardians. Invoke the God by whatever name (or no name) seems good to you, and in the presence of All, bless your stone(s) by air, fire, water, earth, and spirit. Sit quietly before your altar and, with stone in hand, engage in the meditation. Keep your affirmation—to embrace the God and be embraced by Him; to be whole—clearly before you. At the conclusion of the meditation, when it feels right to you, stand before your altar and intone the spell, directing energy into your stone(s) as you do so:

> You step into the moment;
> the sun, like liquid amber,
> covers the afternoon.
> You reach out a hand,
> heavy with the scent of
> honey and almonds,
> to touch my hair.
> You hold the promise of ecstasy
> within the pomegranate's heart;
> if I partake of it I
> will be utterly lost,
> drowning in Your ravishing flood . . .
> take me into the land of rapture;
> liberate the passion You have aroused within.
> My soul longs for union and
> the sweet torrent of release.
> You hold me fast with a lover's kiss;
> Your eyes fill up my sight,
> like an endless desert,
> or like the sun as He covers the moon
> in Her nakedness.
> So mote it be.

When ready, give thanks to All present for Their assistance. Open the Circle and close the Temple.

You may wear your stone in order to you draw God energy to you. You may place it upon your altar as a token of the God. Sleep with it beneath your pillow to dream of Him.

THE TIMING

This spell is best worked on a Sunday at noon, preferably at the height of summer. It may also be worked at the Winter Solstice, as this is a purely God-centered celebration. For the Sacrificed God, Lammas or Samhain are good times, but any time you want to invoke God energy is fine. For the Young Lord growing in strength conduct the meditation during the waxing moon; for the Sacrificed and Dying God the waning moon is best.

THE INCENSE

Cedar, frankincense, myrrh, pine, or sandalwood.

THE CANDLES

Green for the God and gold or red for the fierce light of His energy. Black may be used if you choose to meditate on His sacrificial aspects.

THE PRACTICAL STEPS

- Go to the library and check out some books about mythology. Read some of the stories about the many gods from various cultures. Familiarize yourself with these stories and see how they may have relevance in your life. Often the stories teach about desirable attitudes, deeds, or attributes that the God may embody. How would you incorporate these desirable traits or actions into your life?

- Spend some time in meditation with the God, perhaps in a natural setting where you feel safe and comfortable. Open to Him and allow Him to reveal His face to you. Embrace Him as Mystic Lover, talk to Him as a well-loved friend. Let the experiences come as they may.

- Create an image of the God for your altar through an art project of some sort. Or collect objects that you feel represent the God and place them on your altar. These items may include: acorns, pinecones, select stones, phallic-shaped objects, a bowl of grain, or colorful oak leaves. Let your imagination—and the God—be your guide.

- Pray to the God. Let Him come to you in the ecstasy of prayerful moments. Connect with him in the most sacred space.

- Give some thought to how the men in your life—father, son, lover, spouse—fulfill the various roles of the God for you. Can you see the Divine within these special people? Do you feel differently about them knowing the God may look at you from their eyes? By seeing the Divinity within, you may have a different appreciation for them.

- Pay attention to your dreams. The God may walk with you there, sharing wisdom, offering guidance, or simply revealing His constant and abiding presence.

THE PRIESTESS SPEAKS

The Priestess spoke to a class of acolytes about practicing the presence of the God in their lives. She taught them certain prayers and encouraged them to meditate upon the God. The acolyte went out into the garden. She raised up on tiptoes, lifted her arms, and began a paean of praise to the sun. The warmth of the God's energy enveloped her, and His light embraced her. She was touched by the passion of the God; her eyes glowed.

Part Four

It's Elemental: Working with the Elements

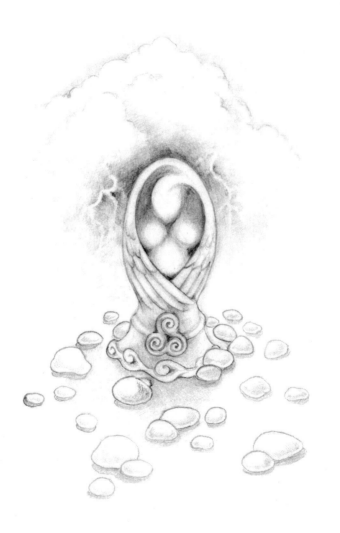

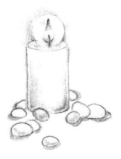

Working with the Elements

*O*nce upon a time, before the world was, the universe was brought forth by the loving attention of the Goddess and the God. In concert They took from Themselves four elements and fashioned from them the earth, the sky, the stars, the waters, and the animal, plant, and mineral kingdoms. From Their knowledge They brought forth air; from Their passion, fire; from Their insight and emotions, water; and from Their creative manifestation, earth. Those elements, plus a fifth, spirit (the joined essence of both), were all that was needed to accomplish Their Great Work.

Every culture from every time has stories about the creation of the universe and all within it, both seen and unseen. A common belief was that the four elements of air, fire, water, and earth were the stuff of creation, with spirit often being the transformative or binding force that energized the others. These elements were within everything and included not only physical properties but mystical ones as well. Eventually they were assigned various attributes, directions, colors, times of the day and of the year, and cycles of the moon, with even plants, animals, gems, and deities attached to them. They were also used in healing, with attempts to understand and treat diseases by balancing these various humors of the body by either adding or subtracting one or more of the elements, often through diet, exercise, and meditation.

Today we know that there are many more than four elements that make up the world. But the mystical properties of the Parent Elements, so crucial to the workings of magic, are fruitful foci for meditation. Through understanding and experiencing Their energies you will become more comfortable working with Them, which will only be helpful in accomplishing your own Great Work.

Air: "To Know"

THE MATERIALS

- A piece of mica large enough and flat enough to use for scrying.

- A yellow pouch made of soft but durable material in which to keep your stone when not in use.

THE PURPOSE

Air. We cannot see it, taste it, grasp it, smell it, or hear it. But it is there, surrounding us and invading and sustaining us with each breath we take. It is invisible and may only be known through its actions: we breathe it in and live. We watch its passage by the dancing of the leaves of the trees. We feel its caress as it breezes past us. Its voice is a whisper, carried to us by the fluttering leaves. It may be soft and gentle or, when roused, terrifying and destructive. Though unseen, it is intimately a part of us and all that lives.

Air has dominion over the east, and thus is called upon for this Quarter when we cast the magic Circle. It stands for rational thought, is logical, and rules the mind and intellectual processes. It represents knowledge and learning. I imagine that all of the great libraries of the world are under the auspices of air. This is a traditionally masculine element. Its time is dawn and its season is spring. The new moon and all new beginnings can be found here.

The magical tools associated with it are the athame and the sword; its symbol is the censor with incense. All flying things, especially birds, are its creatures. Its color is yellow and its planet is Mercury. In some systems the Archangel Raphael is associated with air. Of course, it also rules all winds and breezes, as well as the breath, or life force.

We meditate upon air in order to *know*. We seek to understand our own minds, to think about the work we are doing when we enter our Circle in order to rightly use the power that is available to us. The Delphic oracle encouraged the ancients to "know thyself." This is no less true for us, especially when following any spiritual path.

This spell is for the purpose of flying upon the wings of air in order to gain a better appreciation of our own minds and the intellectual powers that reside within, waiting to be tapped.

THE AFFIRMATION

"I mount air's throne to know myself and rise upon the wings of thought."

THE STONE

Mica forms in thin sheets of crystals that may flake or peel off from each other. It is a rather fragile stone, so be sure and obtain a fairly large piece if you want to work with it. It may be opaque to translucent, depending upon its thickness. The surface is reflective, and traditionally the stone has been used for protection and to reflect back any negative energies. Its brightness and lightness make it appropriate for use in contacting air. Large, flat pieces may be used for scrying, and it is especially appropriate to use for scrying air elementals.

THE GUIDE

The Sylph is an air elemental who may be called upon to guide you through an understanding of this element. He lives upon and within the air, and may be very playful, like an errant breeze. He may have a short attention span, so you need to call upon his name regularly when invoking his presence. He may appear as a beautiful angel surrounded by yellow or golden light with gorgeous wings of peacock blue and the green of hummingbird's wings. Or he may appear in the full glory of a butterfly, or even a golden dragon. Be open to his presence and let him take your hand so that you, too, may experience the joy of flight.

- Air deities include: Enlil (God, Mesopotamian); Su (God, Egyptian); Nut (Goddess, Egyptian); Tatsuta-Hima (Goddess, Japanese).

THE MEDITATION (TO BE DONE IN CIRCLE)

You are a feather floating upon conduits of air. The softest breeze can carry you hither and yon. You enjoy the sensation of simply being, allowing the currents to determine your speed and direction. A very large dragonfly joins you. It shimmers golden in the light, with wings of iridescent blue and yellow. It looks at you curiously and then buzzes you in mid-air! You tumble, end over end, and transform into a beautiful bird. Like the nightingale you have feathers of vibrant color and a long graceful tail. From your throat issues a most beautiful and joyful song, and you dive playfully at the dragonfly. Together you dance upon the air, spinning madly, looping through clouds, then plunging toward the earth only to arise again. You are in your element; air holds no limits or boundaries and you joyfully embrace it with each beat of your wings. The exhilaration of flight opens you up to possibilities; endless streams of thought open out before you, without limits or boundaries. Your soul expands to fill the universe and you see all creation held in the fragile shell of an egg, pregnant with potential.

The dragonfly brings you back to yourself and you gently settle down on a hill. There you see the sky reflected within a piece of mica, and the dragonfly briefly touches it in indication that it is your gift, a reminder of this meditation. You may scry air in this stone at any time and once again be taken by the winds of thought.

THE SPELL

Go to your ritual place. Set up your altar, cast your Circle, and request the presence of the Guardians. Invoke the element air in whatever way seems good to you, and in the presence of All, bless your stone by air, fire, water, earth, and spirit. Sit quietly before your altar and, with stone in hand, engage in the meditation. Keep your affirmation—to mount the throne of air in order to know yourself and to rise upon the wings of thought—clearly before you. At the conclusion of the meditation, when it feels right to you, stand before your altar and intone the spell, directing energy into your stone as you do so:

> Guardian of the east
> Who doth rise upon the Sacred Light,
> You who rides upon the wings of dragons
> and chases the sun from sleep,
> I invoke Your presence here.
> Be my sure guide and lead
> me upon the trackless paths of air.
> You ply the currents of the winds
> and sail beyond the stars,
> and lead me to a deeper
> knowledge of my self.
> "To Know" is Your password.
> Be Thou present now, I pray.
> So mote it be.

When ready, give thanks to All present for Their assistance. Open the Circle and close the Temple.

You may use your piece of mica for purposes of scrying when you need to know something. It may also be placed upon your altar, or used during ritual at the eastern Quarter as a token of air. When not in use keep it in the yellow pouch.

THE TIMING

This spell should be worked on a Wednesday at dawn just after a new moon. Any season is fine in order to meditate on this element, but spring is best, ideally around Imbolc or Ostara.

THE INCENSE

Almond, anise, lavender, lemon, parsley, peppermint, sage, or any "light" smelling incenses or oils you particularly enjoy.

THE CANDLES

Yellow for the element of air.

THE PRACTICAL STEPS

- Meditate upon the element of air, especially in the early morning when the air is fresh. What is it? How does it interact with you on a daily basis. What attributes does it have, and how do these play out in your life? Why is it important to us, to the planet? What does it say to you on a physical level? Or on an emotional, intellectual, and spiritual level? Let the images come.

- Visit the library—a place of knowledge, learning, and the thoughts of deep (and not so deep!) thinkers. Stand in awe and delight at the gifts we have received from these people. Though many are long dead, their words live on for our study and edification. Open a book and open new worlds within.

- Create an art project of some sort depicting air. It may be a collage, a painting, a sculpture, or a weaving. Call upon the Sylphs to help you depict their element. You may be surprised by what you create together.

- Get a wind instrument and play it. Or sing loudly! Let air direct your music and simply enjoy being surrounded by the sound of this element.

- Pay attention to your dreams. Let air speak to you through this mechanism and direct your thoughts. Write down the words and images imparted to you and keep them for future meditations.

THE PRIESTESS SPEAKS

The Priestess sheds her skin and rises into air, a golden bird with crystal song. The acolyte, passing by, drops the basket of herbs she is carrying and watches in disbelief and awe. The golden bird swoops and dives and sings ceaselessly, finally coming to earth, a woman once more. The Priestess, having seen the acolyte, motions the girl to her side with a wink. The acolyte, trembling, stands before her. With one touch the Priestess sends the girl to sleep, to rest among the ferns. There she dreams of golden birds in flight, and dulcet songs of joy.

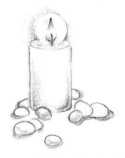

Fire: "To Will"

THE MATERIALS

- A large sunstone.

- A red pouch of soft but durable material in which keep the stone when not in use.

THE PURPOSE

Fire. It dances tamely upon our hearth, or rages out of control, a hungry, angry beast devouring forests and human dwellings alike. It may save life through its warmth or take it in an instant without thought or care. Fire, controlled, heats our homes, cooks our food, and forms metals and minerals into useful objects through its transformative heat. Watch the flames of a fire and it seems like a living thing. Scrying by fire is one way to gaze into the future and uncover truths hiding in the darkness.

Fire has dominion over the south, and thus is called upon for this Quarter when we cast the magic Circle. It stands for action and passion, energy and spirit. This is traditionally a masculine element. Its time is high noon, the hottest time of the day, and its season is summer. The waxing moon, growth, and movement can be found here. The magical tool associated with it is the wand, and candles are its symbol. The dragon that breathes fire is its creature, with the lion and the horse traditionally being assigned to it as well. Its color is red and its planet is Mars. In some systems the Archangel Michael is associated with fire. It also, of course, rules over all types of fire, from the flame on a gas stove to the heaving inferno of an erupting volcano.

We meditate upon fire in order to *will*. We must take thought beyond the realm of air and translate it into action. We seek to tap into our passion in order to allow spirit to rise with the flame of inspiration.

This spell is used for honing our will in the shape of the flame for constructive and life-affirming purposes. We embrace the flame and are purified of all negativity.

THE AFFIRMATION

"I enter the flame, that it may burn away the dross. My will embraces the sacrifice that spirit may burn the brighter."

THE STONE

Sunstone is ruled by the element of fire. There are actually two stones that carry the name. One is a form of quartz with an orange hue, and the other one, known to the ancients and found originally in India, is a type of feldspar. It looks like an orange opal with flecks of hematite embedded within it that cause it to shine and glitter, like sparks of a fire. Traditionally the stone has been used for protection, to promote health and physical energy, and to enhance sexual powers. It is one of the stones related to the God, and, as its name implies, is connected to the sun. It is an appropriate stone to use in your contemplation of fire.

THE GUIDE

The salamander is one of the Guardians of fire, and may be called upon as a guide for your foray into this element. As its name implies, the salamander may appear as a dragonlike being, all in red and gold, with fire edging his wings. Look out, for he breathes fire and also has a short temper! Or he may choose to appear as a young winged warrior with wand or staff in hand, his hair dripping with fire, held back by a golden band. His eyes are of flame, and his hands hot to the touch, yet gentle and able to arouse passionate activity. He will lead you into an inferno of images that will allow you to experience your will.

- Fire deities include: Hephaistos (God, Greek); Tatevali (God, Huichol Indian); Brigid (Goddess, Celtic); Vesta (Goddess, Roman).

THE MEDITATION (TO BE DONE IN CIRCLE)

You stand naked before a winged being of great beauty and power. He is dressed all in hues of red and orange and brilliant yellows. Wings he has, of gold edged in flame. His eyes are soulful, flaming, glorious, and full of promise. He holds out a hand to you dripping with flame, with honey. You take his hand and are immediately swept into an embrace unbearably hot, full of life and energy. Through his eyes you see the world teeming with activity and life. You fearlessly allow him to lead you into the tiny specks of other's life force, and feel the heat generated by their desires and goals and thoughtful activity. Returning to yourself, you recognize that activity ruled by will after careful thought is the only way to reach a goal or accomplish something that is needed. Passion is the fuel to the flame, and only by embracing life in its fullest can passion reign supreme. The fire, in its benign and useful form, is what you seek to nurture in your life. The young salamander, Lord of the Fire, leaves you with a beautiful sunstone. It holds a spark of the flame within its heart and will be a reminder of will-directed activity.

THE SPELL

Go to your ritual place. Set up your altar, cast your Circle, and request the presence of the Guardians. Invoke the element fire in whatever way seems good to you, and in the presence of All, bless your stone by air, fire, water, earth, and spirit. Sit quietly before your altar and, with stone in hand, engage in the meditation. Keep your affirmation—to enter the fire in order to burn away the dross, that through sacrifice your spirit will burn bright—clearly before you. At the conclusion of the meditation, when it feels right to you, stand before your altar and intone the spell, directing energy into your stone as you do so:

> Guardian of the south
> who doth the purifying fire bring,
> You who dance in the flames
> and blaze with the noonday sun,
> I invoke Your presence here.
> Be my sworn guide and lead
> me into the fire's heart.
> Your fierce embrace awakens passion;
> the embers of Your eyes consume me
> and encourage me to
> make my mark upon the world.
> "To Will" is Your password.
> Be Thou present now, I pray.
> So mote it be.

When ready, give thanks to All present for Their assistance. Open the Circle and close the Temple.

You may keep your sunstone with you as a talisman to action. It may be placed upon your altar as a symbol of fire. During ritual it may be placed in the southern Quarter for the same purpose. Gaze into its heart and behold the spark of fire and the life force there.

THE TIMING

This spell should be worked on a Sunday at noon after the moon's first quarter. Any season is fine in order to meditate on this element, but the Summer Solstice is best.

THE INCENSE

Cinnamon, cloves, frankincense, nutmeg, peppermint, sassafras, or tobacco. Any "hot" scent will work fine for this ritual.

THE CANDLES

Red, red, and more red. Get the energy going!

THE PRACTICAL STEPS

- Meditate upon the element fire. Light a candle and simply con-template the flame. As you watch it dance allow your eyes to become unfocused. You will find yourself gazing into the flame's heart. Let it take you where it will.

- Now that you have meditated upon fire, create a list of how it interacts with you in your daily life. With careful thought you may be surprised at how long the list is. Now, give thanks to fire for its many blessings.

- Just as for air, create an art project depicting fire. Let the cre-ative, will-filled aspect of fire inspire you. Use colors and mate-rials that call to you, such as candles, appropriate stones, or bits of red glass. Use a living flame only if you can do so safely. You may also want to create your own wand, since this is a magical tool for this element.

- Pay attention to your dreams. Let fire speak to you through this mechanism and direct your thoughts. Write down the words and images imparted to you and keep them for future meditations.

THE PRIESTESS SPEAKS

The Priestess, teaching a group of acolytes about the element of fire, reaches into the heart of the living flame and begins to fashion it into various forms. The class holds its collective breath, sure she will be burned. The acolyte glances away from what the Priestess is doing and instead gazes into her eyes. She becomes transfixed, for they burn brighter than the fire before them. The Priestess concludes her instruction and says, "Correct honing of the will allows you to accomplish great and wonderful things." She looks right at the acolyte and mirrors the girl's own twin flames with her eyes.

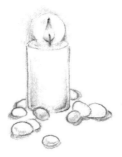

Water: "To Dare"

THE MATERIALS

- A string of pearls.

- A blue pouch of soft but durable material in which to keep the pearls when not in use.

THE PURPOSE

Water covers three-fourths of the earth's surface and is necessary for survival. Without it most forms of life would cease to exist. At its most basic water quenches our thirst, germinates and sustains the seeds as they grow into the food we require, and is used in cooking and cleaning. Its power has been harnessed in order to generate the energy that lights our homes. But water exists independent of our needs and follows its own course. We have all experienced its majesty as we watch it roll onto a beach, restless in its power. Its energy may be felt in the tumbling waterfall or the rushing passage of a river. When one contemplates water one sees beauty and majesty in its changeable depths. The sound of water soothes and refreshes the tired soul. Water is mostly benign toward humans, but when roused it may be highly destructive, taking the form of flooding rivers or lashing rainstorms and hurricanes.

Water has dominion over the west, and thus is called upon for this Quarter when we cast the magic Circle. It represents the power of dreaming, the intuition, and all emotions. Meditation and contemplative prayer are activities in which one may fruitfully engage with this element. This is traditionally a feminine element. Its time is sunset and its season is fall. The waning moon would be found here. The magical tools associated with it are the cauldron and the cup or chalice, both feminine symbols. All water creatures belong to this element, including mermaids, selkies, and nymphs of lake and stream. Its color is blue and its planet is Venus. In some systems the Archangel Gabriel is associated with water. It rules all forms of water, whether free flowing or frozen, and may even be found in steam and mist.

Water may be meditated upon in order to *dare*. Before we may do this, we must dream of the possibilities. Once a dream is embraced we may take steps to reach it. But the unconscious and intuitive process of dreaming is that all-important first step. Sink into the water and envision your future.

THE AFFIRMATION

"Sinking into the water I embrace the dream. Rising, my eyes full of visions, I am ready to dare."

THE STONE

Pearls are formed when a piece of grit or other material is introduced inside the shell of a living creature, an oyster. The oyster, becoming irritated, coats the foreign object with material that hardens and becomes a pearl. Whether saltwater or fresh, the pearl most definitely has an affinity with the element water. Traditionally the pearl has been associated with the moon, and most especially with the Goddess. It has been used in spells for love, abundance, and protection. In harvesting the pearl the animal is killed, thus one must consider carefully the ethical implications of this. For the purpose of this spell, if you do not wish to use real pearls, artificial ones may be substituted. The shape and color of the substitute is sympathetically connected to the real thing and is fine to use, and much kinder to the oyster!

THE GUIDE

Undines are Guardians of the west and of water. They live in this element and may be a perfect guide as you explore the depthless meaning of water. An Undine may appear as a beautiful mermaid, with flashing scales and long gold-green hair. She may appear as a fish, a dolphin, a sea turtle, or any other water creature. She may take the shape of a waterspout or create a body for herself out of crystalline water. She will lead you playfully through this element, but pay attention, for there are meanings within meanings that will flow out before you.

- Water deities are: Aegir (God, Nordic); Poseidon (God, Greek); Tiamat (Goddess, Babylonian); Yemoja (Goddess, Yoruban).

THE MEDITATION (TO BE DONE IN CIRCLE)

You sink into the silence like a stone. The waters embrace you, surround you, submerge you. There is nothing but a sense of lightness. You are suspended between one moment and the next, alive with expectation. Creatures dart about you, small and bright. They are finned and scaled and move with purpose. You follow them. They lead you through fantastic forests of slowly waving kelp and edifices of coral until they part and leave you face-to-face with your guide. The mermaid awaits you and will teach you how to dream. She is beautiful of form, with a powerful tail of blue and rose scales, the flute of gently shaded coral. Her hair is white, and her eyes the ever-changing colors of the sea. She takes your hand and leads you deeper into yourself, taking you to depths you have never reached, to that source of dreaming only partly realized. There you will always find the truth you seek, if you are but wise enough to recognize it. In order to help you she gifts you with a string of pearls, given by consent of the creatures who formed them. You thank them for their sacrifice, and accept their power to return you to the dream-state. Each pearl may hold a vision of what can be, all you must do is dare to follow this vision. The mermaid releases your hand and you gently float to the surface of your current reality, and awaken.

THE SPELL

Go to your ritual place. Set up your altar, cast your Circle, and request the presence of the Guardians. Invoke the element water in whatever way seems good to you, and in the presence of All, bless your stones by air, fire, water, earth, and spirit. Sit quietly before your altar and, with stones in hand, engage in the meditation. Keep your affirmation—to sink into the water and embrace the dream and to rise, ready to dare—clearly before you. At the conclusion of the meditation, when it feels right to you, stand before your altar and intone the spell, directing energy into your stones as you do so:

> Guardian of the west
> who doth cause the sweet waters to flow,
> You who swim the depthless depths
> and receive the sun into His rest,
> I invoke Your presence here.
> Be my sure guide and lead
> me deeper into the hidden realms of water.
> You travel through the currents
> and playfully dance with raindrops,
> and lead me into the depths
> of dreaming, of visions.
> "To Dare" is your password.
> Be Thou present now, I pray.
> So mote it be.

When ready, give thanks to All present for Their assistance. Open the Circle and close the Temple.

You may wear your pearls when settling in for sleep, that they may be a conduit to your dreams. Or they may be placed beneath your pillow. You may put them on your altar to represent water, or during ritual they may be placed at the western Watchtower for the same purpose. Let each shining globe be a reminder to dream, and to dare.

THE TIMING

This spell should be worked on a Friday at sunset during a waning moon. Any season is fine in order to meditate on this element, but the fall is best, ideally around Lammas or the Fall Equinox.

THE INCENSE

Sandalwood.

THE CANDLES

All shades of blue. Some candles may be found with seashells embedded within, and these would be perfect to use on your altar.

THE PRACTICAL STEPS

- Meditate upon the element of water by watching the ocean waves as they roll onto a beach. Try experiencing this at different times of the day, or even at night, in order to see how the changing light affects the mood of the water. Or watch a waterfall as it tumbles from the heights, or a stream as it dances among the rocks. Find a still pool and gaze into it to see what it might yield.

- Create a depiction of water through an art project. You may even use this element in your creation. Such items as shells, water-smoothed stones and glass, driftwood, or depictions of sea creatures may be used. Let this element speak to you and guide your dreaming of this project.

- Submerge yourself in this element. Experience water in its natural state if possible by playing among ocean waves, going river rafting, or boating on a lake. Lacking the ability to do these things, spend some time in a swimming pool or spa, or even simply enjoy a bubble bath. Take a walk in the rain. Let this element speak to you in its many moods, places, and voices.

- This element is strongly connected with dreaming, and may show up more strongly through this avenue. Pay attention to what water says to you in your dreams; let it lead you to dare to live the vision.

THE PRIESTESS SPEAKS

The Priestess takes the acolyte to the Sacred Pool. There she breathes upon the water and invites the girl to seek what it might hold. Sinking into a trance, the acolyte gazes deeply into the pool. The water ripples silently once, then is still. At first the pool simply reflects back to her an image of her face. Then the image flows into colors and shapes so fast the girl cannot tell what they are. Suddenly, the pool turns black. Slowly a vision is reflected back to her. It is her . . . her true self! Water reveals the truth of things. The acolyte is pleased.

Earth: "To Keep Silent"

THE MATERIALS

- A piece of coal.

- A green pouch of soft but durable material in which to keep your stone when not in use.

THE PURPOSE

Earth is the foundation upon which we stand. It is the densest of all the elements. It is slow and steady, weighty and solid. Earth holds all things upon its back. From its rich and fertile substance it brings forth life, and it sustains all life through its bounty. Earth is our Mother in a very real sense, and at the end of life receives us into Her vast womb. Like the other elements, She is our ally, but can be roused to terrible and thunderous activity, causing loss of life and property as She shudders and shakes. We must take care of the earth in order for Her to take care of us. If we do not, we place ourselves, and most especially our posterity, at risk.

Earth has dominion over the north, and thus is called upon for this Quarter when we cast the magic Circle. It stands for manifestation, completion, and the fruit of thought, activity, and dreaming. It is a place of mystery, for before manifestation may occur much is done in silence and is hidden from common eyes. Most Witches' altars face the north. Earth is traditionally a feminine element. Its time is midnight and its season is winter. The dark of the moon just prior to the first sliver of light can be found here. The magical tool associated with it is the pentacle, and its symbol is salt. All creatures that burrow have an affinity with earth, as do those herbaceous beasts who take their life from Her. Gnomes, dwarves, some nymphs and fairies, and other magical folk who understand and work with earth and Her gems, metals, and minerals are also associated with this element. Its color is green and its planet is the earth. In some systems the Archangel Uriel is associated with earth. It rules all forms of earth, including rocks, gems, precious stones, minerals, and metals that are drawn from it, as well as caves and other hidden places.

We meditate upon earth in order to *keep silent.* Just as the seed must lie hidden and quiet before it may sprout to grow into its destiny, so must we learn to keep silent and listen in order for our potential to be realized.

This spell is for the purpose of learning to become silent and to allow the visions, thoughts, and actions we have set in motion to grow to fruition. We become the earth, mysterious and deep, that generates, maintains, and sustains all things in silence.

THE AFFIRMATION

"I enter earth's domain and sink into the silence, that I may grow the seed of tomorrow's aspirations."

THE STONE

Coal is a mineral formed from the partially decomposed remains of vegetable matter kept under great pressure and high temperatures over the course of millions of years. It is combustible and has been used for heating homes and for cooking fires. Being made of vegetable matter and found deep within the earth, it is appropriate to use in this spell. Coal has traditionally been used in prosperity spells and for abundance that we hope to receive from the earth.

THE GUIDE

Gnomes are much more than funny looking plastic statues some people use for lawn decorations! They are creatures of the earth, seemingly formed from out of the earth Herself. They know the secret places and travel the hidden ways. They can unfold the mystery to you. A gnome may appear as a wizened little old lady, or she may appear as a mole, a sow, or other herbivore. She may even choose to reveal herself as a Witch, for the northern Quarter is especially sacred to Witches. In whatever form she may choose, allow her to lead you along the ley lines of the earth to an understanding of this element.

- Earth deities are: Geb (God, Egyptian); Tar (God, Nigerian); Gaia (Goddess, Greek); Tellus (Goddess, Roman).

THE MEDITATION (TO BE DONE IN CIRCLE)

You find yourself in a cavern whose height and breadth and depth you cannot fathom. Living crystals—amethyst, citrine, garnet, and sapphire—glow softly, lighting it steadily, creating rainbows of dancing colors. The deep, rich smell of earth permeates the place and enlivens something within you. There is a sense of things hidden, of sleeping seeds and questing roots all around you. Expectation is in the air. You notice a tunnel stretching out before you and from its inky darkness a diminutive person comes forth. She is dressed in browns and greens, with hair the color of nutmeg and twinkling anthracite eyes. She gives you her name, takes your hand, and leads you into the deeper heart of earth. You become surrounded by a living heartbeat, and as you follow, the gnome begins to uncover earth's secrets. You watch as a seed is placed into the earth. It is small, quiescent, and dreams of *becoming*. It sleeps in silence and is forgotten until, all in a moment, it begins to germinate. Still hidden and unknown, it grows in darkness, keeping its own counsel. Eventually the roots reach deeply, anchoring the seed to life, and the stem stretches upward, ever upward to the light it knows exists until, all unannounced, it breaks the soil and greets the sun. From there it takes but time for it to realize its potential, manifesting fruit or grain or gracious blooms. You are given to understand that all forms of growth may learn from earth; to stay in stillness, to keep silent, to accept the nurturing of others, and to follow one's destiny, like the seed. The gnome, pleased with your understanding, gives you a reminder of your experience: a piece of coal, formed of the earth, to be your future guide.

THE SPELL

Go to your ritual place. Set up your altar, cast your Circle, and request the presence of the Guardians. Invoke the element earth in whatever way seems good to you, and in the presence of All, bless your stones by air, fire, water, earth, and spirit. Sit quietly before your altar and, with stones in hand, engage in the meditation. Keep your affirmation—to enter earth's domain and sink into the silence, that you may grow the seed of tomorrow's aspirations—clearly before you. At the conclusion of the meditation, when it feels right to you, stand before your altar and intone the spell, directing energy into your stones as you do so:

> Guardian of the north
> who doth bless the rich and fertile earth
> and swallow up the midnight sun,
> I invoke Your presence here.
> Be my sure guide and lead
> me through the lightless caverns of earth.
> You know the hidden ways
> and measure time in centuries
> and lead me to the silent places
> of my soul.
> "To Keep Silent" is your password.
> Be Thou present now, I pray.
> So mote it be.

When ready, give thanks to All present for Their assistance. Open the Circle and close the Temple.

You may keep your piece of coal with you as a reminder that sometimes to be in silence is the best place to be. In silence we may hear ourselves, but more importantly we may hear the gods and take counsel with Them. The coal may be placed upon your altar as a representative of earth, or during ritual may be placed at the northern Watchtower for the same purpose. Let it be your guide whenever you enter the silence and reach toward manifestation.

THE TIMING

This spell may be worked on almost any day at midnight during the dark of the moon. Avoid Sunday and Monday. Any season is fine in order to meditate on this element, but winter is best, ideally around Samhain.

THE INCENSE

Bay, cypress, eucalyptus, honeysuckle, patchouli, or any "earthy" scent.

THE CANDLES

Green, from springtime green to deep forest green, for the element of earth.

THE PRACTICAL STEPS

- Meditate on this element. You might want to pick a stone or crystal that calls to you and simply use it as a form to enter this element, or you may wish to sit or lie upon the earth and tune in to the energy you will feel. Let the earth support and cradle you like the Mother She is.

- Create an art project depicting earth. Use pleasing stones, crystals, earth itself, and green and growing things in your creation. Let earth guide you so that you may "grow" something meaningful to you.

- Work in your garden. Let your hands and fingers dig deep into the earth. Let the rich scent of the earth enter into you. Really connect with earth as you work. Cherish the seeds or plants you place within the earth and visualize them growing and becoming.

- If possible spend some time in a cave or cavern. Experience what it is like to be within the womb of earth: the sights, the scents, the feel of the air, the way sound carries or is muffled. Meditate in the darkness and come forth with new insights, with a depth of being that can only come when we drink deep of earth's silence.

THE PRIESTESS SPEAKS

The acolyte, frustrated over her lack of progress on her many projects, is grumpy and out of sorts. The Priestess, seeing this, takes the girl into the sacred cave and tells her to meditate there. Under the earth, within earth's womb, the girl sinks into a trance. There she experiences the slow yet inexorable movement toward completion, toward fruition—of seed, of growing crystal, of the process of decomposition from which new life will form. The acolyte returns to her projects with a sense of patient and quiet activity, knowing that in the fullness of time her "seeds" too would reach completion.

Part Five

Divination with Stones

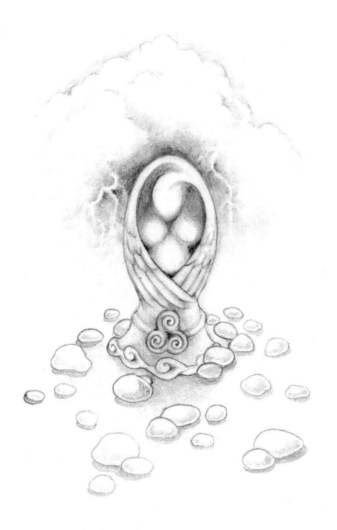

Divination with Stones

*W*ithin precious or semiprecious stones and crystals resides a wealth of knowledge. They have been around for much longer than I have been alive—at least in this incarnation—and I would be foolish not to avail myself of their wisdom. Each stone has its own energy, attributes, and uses. But in the following divinatory practices I have chosen to focus on color as an easy way to connect with the stone's energies. We use color during ritual in order to resonate with those energies we are tapping into, thus using colored stones in divination is one way of receiving hints about the future.

Divination comes from the root word *divine,* which has to do with the Deity. When we utilize forms of divination we are attempting to connect with the Divine Mind in order to receive clarity or guidance about a matter. There are, of course, other ways to do this. One may consult a book, talk with a friend or trained counselor, or in other ways work out the answer to a problem. But if you think that using divination may be of some assistance, the following divinatory casts may be of use. Remember though that the future is not "cast in stone," and that you may always exercise your free will in any matter.

Following is a list of stones and their symbolism. If the colors and their attributes do not fit for you, please feel free to alter them to your needs. Likewise, if I have not mentioned a stone you feel particularly comfortable working with, add it to the list under the appropriate color selection.

There are many divinatory systems available from which to choose, and they will all work, as they tap into the unconscious mind where all answers reside. This system will do the same, whether you use it "as is" or change it to conform more closely to your needs.

For the following divinatory casts you will use just thirteen stones. From the list below, choose one stone from each color selection until you have all thirteen. These will be your working stones. Beneath each heading is the symbolism for that color, which will be used in divining the answers to your questions.

- **Clear stones:** quartz crystal; herkimer diamond; clear tourmaline; clear fluorite.

  Symbolism: clarity of thought; connecting with your HGA (Holy Guardian Angel); physical health and healing.

- **White stones:** moonstone; white marble; howlite; selenite; opal; snowy quartz.

  Symbolism: purification; innocence; the moon; magic; Goddess as Maiden.

- **Yellow stones:** citrine; amber; cat's eye; yellow calcite; yellow jasper; topaz; yellow tourmaline.

  Symbolism: communication; travel; success; leadership; intellectual pursuits; physical energy.

- **Orange stones:** carnelian; sun stone; orange calcite.

  Symbolism: personal power; attraction; movement; stimulation.

- **Red stones:** starry jasper; red jasper; ruby; red garnet; sandstone; cinnabar; red aventurine.

  Symbolism: sexual energy; passion; anger; the heart; change; action; strength; Goddess as Mother.

- **Pink stones:** rhodocrosite; rhodonite; rose quartz; pink agate; pink tourmaline.

Symbolism: romantic love; friendship; joy; relationships; family interaction.

- **Purple stones:** amethyst; sugilite; purple tourmaline.

  Symbolism: connecting with divine energy; the mystical realm; spiritual progress; past lives; prayer; mystical or sacred marriage.

- **Light blue stones:** blue lace agate; aquamarine; blue quartz; blue aventurine; blue fluorite; some turquoise.

  Symbolism: peace; tranquility; discernment; understanding; patience; relieving depression.

- **Dark blue stones:** sodalite; lapis lazuli; azurite; sapphire; blue topaz.

  Symbolism: fidelity; devotion; protection; psychic abilities; dreaming; intuition.

- **Green stones:** amazonite; green aventurine; some turquoise; chrysoprase; malachite; moss agate; peridot; emerald.

  Symbolism: money; prosperity; creativity; growth; fertility; personal goals; abundance; career matters; the Horned God.

- **Brown stones:** tiger-eye; smoky quartz; staurolite (cross stone); fire agate.

  Symbolism: autonomy; inner resources; stability; personal responsibility; grounding.

- **Gray stones:** labradorite; hematite.

  Symbolism: wisdom; knowledge; silence; solitude; simplicity.

- **Black stones:** jet; obsidian; apache tear; black tourmaline; onyx.

  Symbolism: releasing negative energy; binding; receptivity; death; transformation; Goddess as Crone.

As you utilize the following casts allow your intuitive self full rein. Each stone has several meanings, which are represented by a word (for example: red = passion or anger or change). Divine the meaning that is pertinent to your question, then allow the word to sink softly into your unconscious mind. Your intuitive self will take that word and expand upon it, giving you the answer you seek. Simply pay attention and you will have fruitful results.

THIRTEEN STONE CAST

For this cast place all of the stones in a pouch used for the purpose. Hold the pouch while thinking of your question. An example might be, "What do I need to do in order to get the job I want?" Reach into the pouch without looking and draw forth a stone. Place it in front of you. If the answer makes sense to you, stop there; if not, reach in and draw forth another stone. If you are still not sure of the answer, draw a third stone. This will bind the first two. The answers combined will be the answer you seek.

YES/NO CAST

This is used when all you need is a "yes" or "no" answer. While thinking of your question, reach into the pouch and stir the stones around. When you feel the time is right, *lightly* clasp a collection of stones and draw them forth from the pouch. If the number of stones are even, the answer is "yes"; if odd, the answer is "no."

A variation of this is to take a piece of felt and draw a circle on it. Divide the circle in half. On one side write "yes," on the other, write "no." Mark an "x" in the very center of the circle. Hold the pouch while thinking of your question, and when you feel the time is right, tip the bag over the felt circle, making sure to do so over the center point. Then count the number of stones on each side, discarding those sitting on the dividing line or falling outside of the circle. The side with the most stones will be your answer.

SACRED CIRCLE CAST

This is used when you need to know how your past and present will affect a future outcome. Hold the pouch of stones as you ask your question. Next, remove all of the stones from your pouch, one at a time, and place them in a circle (you may use the circle drawn on your felt piece as a guide). Locate the "top" of the circle (the 12:00 position on a clock face). Keeping your question in mind and moving clockwise, pull each fourth stone out of the circle and place it before you, from left to right. Do this until you have three stones in front of you. The leftmost stone is your recent past with regards to the question; the middle stone is the present; and the rightmost stone is the possible future. Read them all together to find your answer.

ELEMENTAL CIRCLE CAST

This is used when you need balance and want to incorporate the wisdom of the elementals into your answer. Place all of the stones in your pouch. As you hold the pouch, think about your question. When ready, reach in and remove one stone. Place this in front of you in the 3:00 position (you may use the circle drawn on your felt piece for a guide). This is the stone for the element of the east, which is air and is concerned with your thoughts and intuition about the matter. Reach in the pouch and remove another stone. This will be placed in the 6:00 position and is the stone for the element of the south, which is fire. This stone is concerned with your will and actions. Now remove a third stone and place it in the 9:00 position. This is the stone for the element of the west, which is water, and is concerned with your emotions and feelings about the matter. Draw out a fourth stone and place it at the 12:00 position. This is the stone for the element of the north, which is earth, and is concerned with manifesting results. Finally, draw out a fifth stone and place it in the center. This is the stone for spirit, which is everywhere. It is concerned with transformation and change, and of the Divine Mind.

Now starting with air and moving around the circle, discern what each stone is telling you about each aspect of the question. The spirit stone may be a clarification of the answer by tying all of the other answers together.

CHAKRA MEDITATION

This is a meditation rather than a divinatory exercise, yet it may also be used to locate areas of physical concern or stress.

Choose seven stones with colors to represent each of the seven chakras. They should be laid out as follows:

7 = Crown chakra: amethyst or violet (white)*

6 = Third Eye or Brow chakra: dark blue or indigo (amethyst)*

5 = Throat chakra: light blue

4 = Heart chakra: green

3 = Solar Plexus chakra: yellow

2 = Naval chakra: orange

1 = Root chakra: red

Once your stones are laid out, pick up the first stone, for the Root chakra, and hold it in your dominant hand. Close your eyes, meditate on the color red, and visualize your Root chakra opening like a lotus flower. When it feels as if it is fully open, move on to the next stone and the next chakra. If there are any blockages along the way you might feel it in your body at that chakra point, or in the stone you are holding. Pay special attention to that area. Once all of the chakras are open, simply sit in quiet meditation, drawing health and balance to yourself. When you feel the time is right, close each chakra, beginning at the Crown and moving down to the Root, visualizing each energy point closing up like the petals of a flower. This is a good meditation to use for balance and inner healing.

---

* In some systems the Crown chakra is imaged as bright white, while the Third Eye or Brow chakra is imaged as amethyst. You may use these colors if you wish.

The worksheet below may be used to keep a record of the questions you ask, their answers, your interpretation, and any actions you may need to take as a response.

Question:
Answer:
Interpretation:
Action:

Part Six

Using Meditation Beads

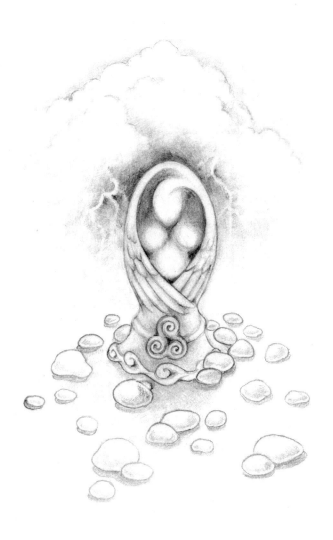

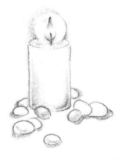

Communing with the Goddess and the God

Thirteen moons upon a
silver chain;
the Goddess, triple-formed,
a radiant crown.
Prayers drip like honey,
or morning's milky dew,
as holy approbation
becomes our benison.

—GALEN GILLOTTE

The cool beads slip effortlessly through your fingers. The murmur of prayers accompanies the movement from one bead to another. Everything around you recedes as your spirit flows into word and action and expands with an open heart, awaiting the touch of the Goddess and the God.

Prayer beads of some sort have been used in various religious practices for thousands of years. They have been used as a counting mechanism, to remind the faithful how many of a prescribed number of prayers have been said. They have been used for purposes of meditation, to help focus the mind and heart upon the Deity. The beads themselves are not magic; they are used as an aid for meditational and devotional practices, such as (and especially) the repetition of prayers or the repetition of a name of a god or goddess. These devotions and meditations become a lens through which union with the Deity may occur.

The Wiccan community, those who follow the Wheel of the Year and the Dance of the Goddess and the God, is in need of devotional practices that will aid in opening the door to the Sacred. Magic, spells, and rituals have always been a part of the Pagan path, but for the quiet soul who seeks union with Deity, other forms may be needed and/or desired. Here I offer the idea and use of meditational prayer beads as a path to holiness and the wholeness that results from sacred union.

The origin of beads for purposes of prayer is lost in antiquity. Almost every religious culture seems to have found a use for them in keeping count or "telling" prayers, and often the idea was borrowed by one religious tradition from another.

According to author Lois Sherr Dubin (*The History of Beads from 30,000 B.C. to the Present*), the word "bead" comes from the Anglo-Saxon *bidden,* meaning "to pray," and *bede,* meaning "prayer." Thus saying one's beads simply meant saying one's prayers. Since there were usually a certain number of prayers for the faithful to say, beads were eventually used to help illiterate members keep track of how many prayers were completed. It was only later that their use for meditation was added in some traditions. The beads also offered a tactile experience that was an aid in keeping errant thoughts on the task at hand and establishing a kinesthetic memory, thus strengthening the habit of prayer.

In her history of beads, Dubin traced the use of prayer beads through a variety of centuries. Though they are most strongly associated with the West and Roman Catholicism, they actually had their origin in the East prior to the founding of Christianity. Hindus may have been the first people to utilize this prayer form (possibly around 600 B.C.E.), and it is still found in that tradition today. Hindu prayer beads, called *mala,* meaning "garden," or *japamala,* meaning "rose chaplet," are comprised of either 108 beads for followers of the god Vishnu, or thirty-four or sixty-four beads, used by followers of the god Shiva. For the devout Hindu the beads are told morning, noon, and night, with the *mala* held over the stomach, heart, and nose, respectively. The beads are placed in a bag, with the right hand and fingers manipulating the beads while the beads themselves remain out of sight. Most mala are made of wood, with devotees of Vishnu carrying beads made of rudrsksha seeds, while those of Shiva are made out of the tulsi, or holy basil, tree.

The Buddhists probably borrowed the idea of prayer beads from the Hindus (around 500 B.C.E.), and when Buddhist monks carried the teaching of Buddha's Middle Path to Tibet, China, Japan, and other areas, they were adopted by those cultures. Buddhist prayer beads differ in number and type of prayers depending upon the type of Buddhism practiced. Indian and Tibetan Buddhist strands are comprised of 108 beads, though the latter divide their sets into four groups of twenty-seven beads. Japanese Buddhist beads, called *sho-zoiki jiu-dzu,* are comprised of 112 beads and refer to different gods and saints. Wood is the preferred material for Japanese and Indian beads, while Tibetan beads could be made from any material, including precious gems, they were held in such high esteem.

Islamic beads, called *subha,* meaning "to exalt," were probably borrowed from the Buddhists. Their strands are comprised of ninety-nine beads for the ninety-nine names of Allah, and may be made of wood, shells, or precious and semiprecious stones.

Christianity probably got the idea for prayer beads from the Muslims when exposed to this prayer form during the Crusades, but this is by no means certain. The rosary, from the Latin *rosarium,* meaning "rose garden," was attributed to St. Dominic (1170–1221), but there seems to be no historical evidence for this. In fact, some form of the rosary was in use as early as 366 C.E., and was mentioned by St. Augustine.

The rosary was originally used to keep track of a prescribed number of prayers. The psalms, which number 150, were often memorized by members of religious communities and counted off bead by bead. Later, the *Pater Noster* (or the "Our Father") was repeated on the beads. Finally, a combination of the *Ave Maria* (or "Hail Mary") and the "Our Father" was counted, with other prayers added as time passed.

The modern rosary is made up of fifty-nine beads, with five groups of ten beads that are divided by additional beads. Prescribed prayers are said upon each bead, and since around the sixteenth century, meditations have been attached to the use of these beads. These fifteen "Mysteries" are scenes from the lives of Jesus and Mary. They are: the five Joyful Mysteries, the five Sorrowful Mysteries, and the five Glorious Mysteries. As these meditational scenes were embraced, the rosary became more than simply a mechanism for keeping track of the number of prayers said; it became an aid to deepen one's spiritual prayer life.

The Greek Orthodox Church also uses a form of rosary called the *kombologion*. It is a knotted rosary made of cord, and has been unchanged since the earliest days of Christianity. It was conferred upon the newly-made monk and to this day is called his "spiritual sword."

Prayer beads were, and are, made of many materials, from humble wood, seeds, and shells to precious and semiprecious stones such as jade, pearls, amber, rubies, and emeralds. At times they were used not only for devotional purposes, but also as jewelry and as a way of impressing others with one's wealth.

All of the prayer beads previously discussed have one unifying feature in spite of the differing numbers of beads, variety of forms, and credos: the arrangement of the beads into a circle.

Wiccans have recognized the sacredness of the circle for time out of mind. We use it in our rituals and, once cast, it creates a boundary between the worlds that allows us to build and maintain energy that may be used for various purposes. The circle has also been used as a symbol of protection. According to Scott Cunningham, it ". . . represents the Goddess, the spiritual aspects of nature, fertility, infinity, eternity. It also symbolizes the Earth itself" (Cunningham 1988, 59). Psychologically it represents wholeness, completion, perfection, the cycle of life and death. The Wheel of the Year, marked by the "beads" of the sacred holy days, is yet another form of the circle, where beginnings beget endings and endings are but illusion.

Prayer beads, then, represent all of these things. Though held in the hand, they form a circle of silent and solitary prayer, drawing the soul into communion with her beloved, ringing both into intimate union.

Telling Your Beads: For the Goddess

In holy silence we seek the altar of the
Goddess, and become absorbed in prayers of
breathless adoration.

—GALEN GILLOTTE

You may use your beads whenever and wherever you wish. They are made to be portable and, once you commit the simple prayers to memory, can be used to fill in those odd free moments with prayer. Your beads may be used for several purposes. The following are some of them, though you may find others.

In order to use the prayer beads for meditation and union with the Goddess, you may want to seek out silence and solitude, and take the contemplative attitude of quiet waiting as you say your prayers. The meditational aspect comes in when you become so absorbed in the telling of the prayers that they seem to tell themselves, and your soul crosses the boundaries of the world to a place that is elsewhere, with the Goddess, in that realm of perfect union and completion.

You may also use the beads to focus energy towards some goal. For example, you may say the beads for the purpose of getting a good job, bringing love into your life, or enhancing some quality you would like more of, such as compassion, generosity, or patience. They may also be said for the purpose of gaining strength to cope with some difficulty in your life. As you say your beads, focus on your intention, and as you say the final prayer, release the energy so that your purpose may be realized.

Another wonderful use for the beads is to simply count your blessings. This helps to replace negative thoughts with positive ones, and reinforces the habit of seeing the good in your life, and it helps you to maintain balance.

You may also use your beads with others. Group prayer is very powerful, and the act of engaging in verbal prayer with others will aid you in your own spiritual growth. You will be surprised at the energy raised if this manner of prayer is practiced, and at your sense of union, not only with Goddess, but with your sister prayers as well.

The primary purpose of the beads, as I see it, is to be drawn into closer union with Goddess. One way of drawing closer is to meditate upon each aspect of Her as you say the beads. Her triple aspect of Maiden-Mother-Crone is full of rich symbolism and will give you much in the way of meditational material. The appendix offers some insights into the Triple Goddess to get you started.

Following are the prayers that are to be said while saying your beads. Please refer to Figure 1, "For the Goddess," and Figure 2, "For the God," to see which bead carries which prayer. The instructions to construct your prayer beads follow the prayers. May your own personal garden of prayers encircle you with the light of the Goddess and the God, and may Their love fill you with the sweet fragrance of holiness. Blessed be.

PRAYERS FOR THE GODDESS

Opening Prayer

In the temple of the moon
by air, fire, water, earth
let my prayers rise unto Thee
in wonder and in mirth.
Blessed be.

For the Maiden*

Hail Bright Maiden of quicksilver delight,
shine upon me Thy blessing which,
like the new dawn, refreshes my spirit and
lifts my heart with song.
Blessed be.

For the Mother*

Hail Mother of the golden wheat, You of
plenty and fertile womb, breathe Thy blessing
upon my heart; nourish my soul that I,
too, may create the world with love.
Blessed be.

For the Crone*

Hail Dark Lady of the crossroads, of wisdom
hard won, grant me Thy blessing, purify my
heart, and teach me the truth of my soul;
show me that death is but the gateway to life.
Blessed be.

Self-Blessing*

By air and by fire
I am blessed.
By water and by earth
I am blessed.
By sprit I am blessed.
Lord and Lady, bless me.
Blessed be.

---

* These prayers may be found in some form in *Book of Hours: Prayers to the Goddess*.

For the Lady

Lady bless me.
Lady keep me.
Lady light my way.
In life and death
You are my hope
so hold me in Your heart
I pray.
Blessed be.

Closing Prayer

Lady,
I give Thee thanks
for Thy many blessings and
hopes fulfilled.
In perfect love and
perfect trust
I adore and honor Thee.
Blessed be.

THE MATERIALS

- For the lead piece, a representative charm of the Goddess, a stone worked into the likeness of the full moon, or a clear quartz, amethyst, or rose quartz crystal with either a hole drilled through the top or a small ring attached to it for fastening.

- For the next piece, a pentacle with attachments at the top and bottom, or a pleasing bead drilled through.

- Thirty-nine drilled beads from 12 mm. to 14 mm. in size. You may use pearls, faux pearls (in order to obtain real pearls, the oyster must die, so faux pearls may be used in their stead), moonstones, amethysts, clear quartz, jet, amber, bone (if you can be assured that the animal's death was humane), or any stone that speaks to you of Goddess.

- Three drilled beads, a little larger than the others. One to represent the Goddess in Her Maiden aspect, such as clear quartz; one for Her Mother aspect, such as amethyst or amber; and one for Her Crone aspect, such as jet or moonstone. They may be the same as the others or each may be different.

- Cord, embroidery floss, or other material on which you can string the beads.

- Needle of an appropriate size.

- A pouch in which to keep your meditation beads (the "witchier" the better).

- Assemble the beads as shown in Figure 1 (page 260), then utilize the prayers as noted.

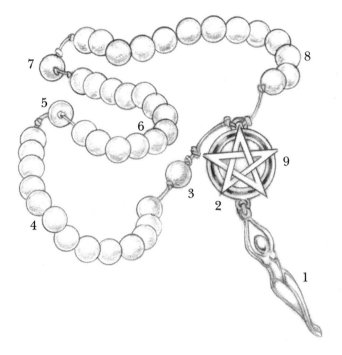

Figure 1: For the Goddess

1. Opening Prayer (on the Goddess bead or crystal)

2. Self-Blessing (on the pentacle or other appropriate stone)

3. For the Maiden (on the first large bead)

4. For the Lady (on the first set of thirteen moons)

5. For the Mother (on the second large bead)

6. For the Lady (on the second set of thirteen moons)

7. For the Crone (on the third large bead)

8. For the Lady (on the third set of thirteen moons)

9. Closing Prayer (said at the end)

Telling Your Beads: For the God

The God in silence
walks the land,
in silence does
he hunt—
a silver swan;
an ivory doe—
all flee before the sun.
He hunts by scent,
by sight, by sound,
this Hunter of the Night.
He hunts me now,
He's on my trail,
and pledges sweet delight.

—GALEN GILLOTTE

The Horned God is an integral, and intimate, half to the whole that is Deity. He partners the Goddess around the Wheel of the Year; He is born of Her, courts Her, enters into the Sacred Marriage with Her, impregnates Her, and dies—sometimes at Her hands—so that we may live and flourish. The Goddess takes Him into Her womb again, and the cycle starts anew.

The meditation beads for the God may be used in the same way as those for the Goddess. They may be used simply for closer union with the God, for the purpose of focusing upon a goal, to show your gratitude to Him and to count your blessings, and to use during group prayer.

While meditating upon the God may you encounter His strength, energy, eroticism, laughter, devotion, love, mischief, and glory.

PRAYERS TO THE GOD

Opening Prayer
In the temple of the sun
by fire, water, earth, and air,
let my prayers rise unto Thee
and teach my soul to dare.
Blessed be.

*Self-Blessing**
By air and by fire
I am blessed.
By water and by earth
I am blessed.
By sprit I am blessed.
Lord and Lady, bless me.
Blessed be.

For the Horned God
Lord of woods and
field and streams,
hunter of the moon
and keeper of the dream,
by stem and leaf
and golden grain,

---

* This prayer may be found in some form in *Book of Hours: Prayers to the Goddess.*

I seek Your blessing;
I call Your name.
Blessed be.

Closing Prayer

Lord,
I give Thee thanks
for Thy many blessings and
hopes fulfilled.
In perfect love and
perfect trust
I adore and honor Thee.
Blessed be.

THE MATERIALS

- For the lead piece, a representative charm of the Horned God, a stone fashioned into the sun, or a clear quartz or citrine crystal.

- For the next piece, a pentacle with fasteners on top and bottom, or a pleasing bead, drilled through.

- Twenty-one drilled stones from 12 mm. to 14 mm. in size. Appropriate stones include sun stone, moss agate, carnelian, tiger-eye, citrine, bone or antler (if you can be assured that the animal's death was humane), or any other stone that speaks to you of the God.

- Cord, embroidery floss, or other appropriate material on which to string them.

- Needle of an appropriate size.

- A pouch in which to keep them that is made of woodland green, brown, gold, or red.

- Assemble the beads as shown in Figure 2 (page 264), then utilize the prayers as noted.

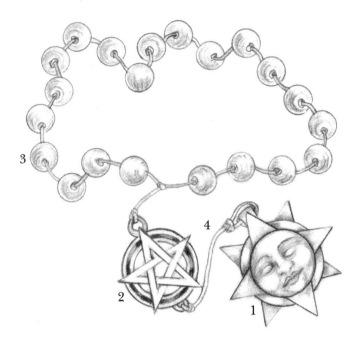

Figure 2: For the God

1. Opening Prayer (on the God bead or crystal)

2. Self-Blessing (on the pentacle or other appropriate stone)

3. For the Horned God (on the set of twenty-one beads)

4. Closing Prayer (said at the end)

Prayer beads are not magic. They have a long and rich history of use by many cultures and religious traditions, and may be a powerful door to holiness and that most desired union with Deity. If you have the desire to pray and meditate, placed there by the Goddess and the God, pick up your beads and let them help you. They may just take you to a place you have been dreaming of: they may just take you home.

Afterword

*Y*ou have now experienced meditation and magic for everyday living in your own life. Through the use of your intellect, your passion, your hard work and talents, your ability to dream, and your willingness to surrender to the process, you have spun your dreams into reality. You have opened to possibilities, greeted the Goddess in many of Her guises, and made powerful allies of crystals and stones whose untapped energies awaited your touch. By using some of the spells in this book you have engaged the arts of meditation and magic on your own behalf, and along the way have learned some new skills, become more insightful, touched your creativity into being, connected with nature and the gods, or deepened your connection and commitment to yourself and others. Through your own efforts you have gained your heart's desires.

Magic is everywhere. It rides upon the night sky, an ivory tower made of light. It speaks with the sea's voice. It clamors for attention in the lushness of blossom and fruit. It looks at you from the clear eyes of a child. There is no trick to magic; simply be open to it and believe.

May your dreams find their way to you in the fullness of their manifestation.

So mote it be.

Appendix

For those who wish to utilize God-energy in the spells of this book, the following is a list of God-aspects to address and connect with. There are many excellent books to look into in order to deepen your knowledge and understanding of these aspects, many of which may be found in the reference section that follows. Explore those aspects you wish to use until you can visualize them fully and move them into the meditations.

If you are a man utilizing these spells, alter the meditations to better fit your needs. The spells are for all, and are fluid enough to live in your unconscious in the manner that will work best for you.

- To discover your spiritual path: Buddha (India); Krishna (India); Jesus Christ (Semitic).

- For the home: Lo'cin-coro'mo (Siberian); Penates (Roman); Zao-jun (Chinese).

- To increase magical abilities: Nuada (Celtic); Kompera (Japanese); Kanaloa (Hawaiian).

- For maintaining health: Apollo (Greek); Aesculapius (Greek); Belenus (Celtic).

- To obtain clarity: Logos (Greek); Ganesha (Indian); Merlin (Celtic).

- To draw love into your life: Amor (Roman); Manmatha (Indian); Pradyumna (Indian).

- For fidelity: Adonis (Greek); Demuzi (Mesopotamian); Fides (Roman).

- For creative chaos: Gobniu (Celtic); Ptah (Egyptian); Apsu (Babylonian); Coyote (Native American).

- For friendship: Airyaman (Persian); Mithra (Iranian); Wadd (pre-Islamic Southern Arabian).

- For peace: Freyr (Norse); Janus (Roman); Olorun (Yoruban).

- To enhance communication: Ogmius (Celtic); Vagisvara (Buddhist); Papa Legba (Haitian).

- For purification: Februus (Etruscan); Izanagi (Japanese).

- For autonomy: Sarutahiko Ohkami (Japanese).

- To increase wisdom: Enli (Mesopotamian); Ganesha (Indian); Thoth (Egyptian).

- For abundance: Bagisht (Afghan); Dedwen (Nubian); Kubera (Indian).

- For success: Eventus Bonus (Roman).

- For justice: Pao Kung (Chinese); Rasnu (Persian); Samas (Mesopotamian); Thor (Norse).

- For transformation: Vertumnus (Roman).

- For protection: Cheng-huang (Chinese protection deities); Balam (Mayan protection deities).

- To accept the cycles of our lives: Cernunnos (Celtic); Adon (Phoenician).

- To increase a parent's love: Fabulinus (Roman); Pilumnus (Roman).

- To connect with your inner child: Pan (Greek); Krishna (as a boy, Indian).

- To promote dreaming: Morpheus (Greek).

- For confronting death: Anubis (Egyptian); Hades (Greek); Thanatos (Greek).

- For rebirth: Kukulcan (Mayan); Shou-Xing (Chinese); Osiris (Egyptian); Jesus Christ (Semitic).

MOON PHASES AND THEIR MEANINGS

Part of conducting successful spells is a consideration of the timing. The major aspect of timing has to do with the moon and Her phases.

New Moon

This is the time when the moon is but a slender sliver in the night sky. She emerges from the darkness, showing Her small light in token of new hopes and new beginnings. Starting anything that moves toward growth and increase at this time is highly advantageous.

Waxing Moon

This is the time when the moon is growing from new to full. As the nights pass, you can see Her grow toward ripe roundness as Her light steadily increases. It is appropriate at this time to begin or continue those spells that move toward increase and fullness.

Full Moon

This is the time when the moon is full and pregnant and rides the night sky in splendor, shedding Her light and beneficence upon all. At this time we see a completion of those spells begun at new moon, or anytime during Her waxing phase. This is also traditionally the time that Witches meet to celebrate the Goddess, and is a time of power and mystery. The celebration may include the day before, the day of, and the day after the full moon in order to encompass the Goddess in Her aspects of Maiden, Mother, and Crone.

Waning Moon

This is the time when the moon begins to decrease in size, scope, and brightness until She disappears from sight. During this phase spells dealing with binding, releasing, or decreasing are conducted.

Dark of the Moon

This is the time when the moon is hidden from our sight, trembling upon the edge of return into the night. Many Witches do not do magic at this time, but rather rest and contemplate. The dark of the moon is full of mystery and magic; it may offer fruitful meditations about issues of death, loss, transformation, and the thought that goes into the planting of seeds of our future desires.

THE TIMING

The phases of the moon are just one way of determining when a spell should be conducted. The days of the week are also to be taken into consideration, as they have traditionally been allocated various characteristics, with different tasks assigned depending upon what one wants to accomplish. Following are just some suggestions. You will note that in some cases a task has been assigned to more than one day of the week. There are subtle influences that each offers, and a spell may work well on more than one day, depending upon the nuance one wishes to utilize.

- Monday: spirituality; home; magic; relationships; fidelity; peace; cycles; parental love; dreaming and visions; menopause; reincarnation; birth; initiation; Goddess.

- Tuesday: autonomy; strength; courage.

- Wednesday: creativity; communication; wisdom; intelligence; air.

- Thursday: abundance; success; justice and legal matters; leadership; power; responsibility; business activities.

- Friday: love; relationships; friendship; physical pleasure; sexuality; water.

- Saturday: home; magic; purification; wisdom; transformation; menopause; time; death.

- Sunday: health and healing; clarity; confidence; peace; autonomy; protection; inner child; joy; God; fire.

THE TRIPLE GODDESS

The Maiden

The Maiden is the innocent, virgin aspect of the Goddess, symbolized by the new moon. She represents all things new: beginnings, projects, attitudes, relationships, changes, and so on. When we are weary, She is the one to connect with in order to seek renewal. Her color is white.

The Mother

The Mother is the fertile, fecund, creative aspect of the Goddess, symbolized by the full moon. She represents growth, increase, generosity, abundance, prosperity, rebirth, and compassion. She is the One to connect with when we wish to be creative and to understand and accept our interconnection with all others, as well as the various caregiving roles we may have in our lives. Her color is red.

The Crone

The Crone is the empty, dark, receptive, and destructive aspect of the Goddess, symbolized by the dark of the moon. She represents waiting, stillness, silence, death, decrease, destruction, loss, and grief. She is also goddess of mystery, magic, passages, and transformative power. She is the One to connect with when we wish to move beyond obstacles or barriers, or when we require wisdom to understand a situation that we are going through. With destruction and loss comes room for new growth and beginnings, and often this aspect leads us right back to the Maiden. Her color is black.

HOUSE BLESSING

After you have cast your Circle, invoked the Guardians, and invited the Goddess and the God to be present, take the incense, then light and bless it by saying:

> Blessed be thou, O creature of air.
> Blessed by thou, O creature of fire.
> [Thus you have the elements of air and fire in the incense censor.]

Take a bowl, pour water into it, add salt, and bless it by saying:

> Blessed be thou, O creature of water.
> Blessed by thou, O creature of earth.
> [Thus, combined in the bowl, are the elements of water and earth.]

Cut a doorway into the Circle, then take the incense censor in one hand, and the bowl in the other (be sure to close the Circle after you exit it). Starting at the front door and working through the house clockwise, bless all the doors, windows, and any other openings to your home in the following manner:

> In the name of the Goddess and the God
> by air and by fire I banish all negative influences
> from this house.
> [Make the sign of a banishing pentagram with the censer].
> By water and by earth I banish all negative influences
> from this house.
> [Make the sign of a banishing pentagram with the bowl].
> Be gone! Be gone! Be gone away!
> Let only light, life, love, and laughter enter herein.

When the circuit of the house is complete, return to the altar. Visualize the protective Circle expanding to the perimeters of the property you hold in trust for the Goddess and the God. Visualize a Cone of Power encircling the boundaries, and light flooding your Sacred Space.

When done, give thanks, earth the power in the usual manner, open the Circle, and close the Temple.

References

BEADS: PRAYER ASPECTS

Dubin, Lois Sherr. 1987. *The History of Beads from 30,000 B.C. to the Present.* N.Y.: Harry N. Abrams, Inc., Publishers.

Erickson, Joan Mowat. 1969. *The Universal Bead.* N.Y.: W. W. Norton & Company Inc.

Filstrup, Chris and Janie. 1982. *Beadazzled: The Story of Beads.* N.Y.: Frederick Warne & Co., Inc.

Harper, Howard V. 1957. *Days and Customs of All Faiths.* N.Y.: Fleet Publishing Corporation.

Cavendish, Richard, ed-in-chief. 1983. *Man, Myth & Magic: The Illustrated Encyclopedia of Mythology, Religion and the Unknown.* (Psych-Skin). N.Y.: Marshall Cavendish.

———. (Time-Zurv). 1983. N.Y.: Marshall Cavendish.

Wilkinson, Philip. 1999. *Illustrated Dictionary of Religions: Figures, Festivals, and Beliefs of the Worlds' Religions.* N.Y.: DK Publishing, Inc.

DEITIES

Ardinger, Barbara. 1999. *Goddess Meditations.* St. Paul, Minn.: Llewellyn Publications.

Conway, D. J. 1997. *Lord of Light and Shadows: The Many Faces of the God.* St. Paul, Minn.: Llewellyn Publications.

Gillotte, Galen. 2002. *Book of Hours: Prayers to the God.* St. Paul, Minn.: Llewellyn Publications.

———. 2001. *Book of Hours: Prayers to the Goddess.* St. Paul, Minn.: Llewellyn Publications.

Hunt, Lisa. 2001. *Celestial Goddesses.* St. Paul, Minn.: Llewellyn Publications.

Jordan, Michael. 1993. *Encyclopedia of Gods: Over 2,500 Deities of the World.* N.Y.: Facts on File, Inc.

Farrar, Janet, and Stewart Farrar. 1987. *The Witches' Goddess.* Custer, Wash.: Phoenix Publishing, Inc.

———. 1989. *The Witches' God.* Custer, Wash.: Phoenix Publishing, Inc.

Imel, Martha Ann, and Dorothy Myers. 1993. *Goddesses in World Mythology: A Biographical Dictionary.* N.Y.: Oxford University Press.

Monaghan, Patricia. 1999. *The Goddess Path: Myths, Invocations and Rituals.* St. Paul, Minn.: Llewellyn Publications.

———. 2000. *The New Book of Goddesses and Heroines.* St. Paul, Minn.: Llewellyn Publications.

Shinoda Bolen, M.D., Jean. 1984. *Goddesses in Everywoman: A New Psychology of Women.* N.Y.: Harper & Row, Publishers.

Stassinopoulos, Agapi. 1999. *Conversations with the Goddesses: Revealing the Diving Power Within You.* N.Y.: Stewart, Tabori & Chang.

Telesco, Patricia. 1998. *365 Goddess: A Daily Guide to the Magic and Inspiration of the Goddess.* N.Y.: Harper Collins Publisher, Inc.

Trobe, Kala. 2000. *Invoke the Goddess: Visualizations of Hindu, Greek and Egyptian Deities.* St. Paul, Minn.: Llewellyn Publications.

Walker, Barbara G. 1983. *The Woman's Encyclopedia of Myths and Secrets.* N.Y.: Harper Collins Publisher, Inc.

MAGIC

Crowley, Aleister. 1976. *Magick: In Theory and Practice.* N.Y.: Dover Publications, Inc.

———. *The Book of the Law.* 1976. (Privately issued by the O.T.O.). N.Y.: Samuel Weiser.

Cunningham, Scott. 1988. *Wicca: A Guide for the Solitary Practitioner.* St. Paul, Minn.: Llewellyn Publications.

Hawke, Elen. 2000. *In the Circle: Crafting the Witches' Path.* St. Paul, Minn.: Llewellyn Publications.

Starhawk. 1979. *The Spiral Dance: A Rebirth of the Ancient Religion of the Great Goddess.* San Francisco: Harper & Row, Publishers.

MEDITATION

Cori, Jasmin Lee. 2000. *The Tao of Contemplation: Re-sourcing the Inner Life.* York Beach, Maine: Samuel Weiser, Inc.

Da, Liu. 1986. *T'ai Chi Ch'uan and Meditation.* N.Y.: Schocken Books.

Galenhorn, Yasmine. 1997. *Trancing the Witch's Wheel: A Guide to Magickal Meditation.* St. Paul, Minn.: Llewellyn Publications.

Monaghan, Patricia, Diereck Monaghan, and G. Eleanor. 1999. *Meditation: The Complete Guide.* Novato, Calif.: New World Library.

Nhat Hanh, Thich. 1975. *The Miracle of Mindfulness: A Manual on Meditation.* Boston, Mass.: Beacon Press.

Roche, Lorin. 1998. *Meditation Made Easy.* N.Y.: HarperSanFrancisco/HarperCollins Publishers.

MISCELLANEOUS

Bowes, Susan. 1999. *Life Magic: The Power of Positive Witchcraft.* N.Y.: Simon & Schuster.

Cunningham, Scott. 1982. *Magical Herbalism: The Secret Craft of the Wise.* St. Paul, Minn.: Llewellyn Publications.

———. 2000. *The Complete Book of Incense, Oils and Brews.* St. Paul, Minn.: Llewellyn Publications.

New American Bible. 1976. Iowa Falls, Iowa: World Bible Publishers.

Our Bodies, Ourselves for the New Century: A Book by and for Women.
May, 1998. Boston Women's Health Collective. Touchstone
Books. Revised and updated edition.

Slater, Herman, ed. 1974–1975. *A Book of Pagan Rituals.* York
Beach, Maine: Samuel Weiser, Inc.

Webster's New Twentieth Century Dictionary, Unabridged. 1983. N.Y.:
Simon & Schuster.

STONES

Conway, D. J. 1999. *Crystal Enchantments: A Complete Guide to Stones
and Their Magical Properties.* Freedom, Calif.: The Crossing Press.

Cunningham, Scott. 1998. *Cunningham's Encyclopedia of Crystal,
Gem and Metal Magic.* St. Paul, Minn.: Llewellyn Publications.

Duda, Rudolf, and Tubos Rejl. 1986. *Minerals of the World.* N.Y.:
Arch Cape Press.

Hall, Judy. 2000. *The Illustrated Guide to Crystals.* N.Y.: Sterling
Publishing Company, Inc.

Medici, Mariana. 1988. *Good Magic.* N.Y.: Prentice Hall Press.

Pough, Frederick, H. 1976. *A Field Guide to Rocks and Minerals.* 4th
ed. Boston, Mass.: Houghton Mifflin Company.

Simpson, Liz. 1997. *The Book of Crystal Healing.* N.Y.: Sterling
Publishing Co., Inc.

Walker, Barbara G. 1989. *The Book of Sacred Stones: Fact and Fallacy
in the Crystal World.* N.Y.: HarperCollins Publishers.